Review
of **Pediatrics**

Review
of Pediatrics

FOURTH EDITION

RICHARD D. KRUGMAN, M.D.

Professor of Pediatrics
Dean, University of Colorado
School of Medicine
Director, The C. Henry Kempe National
Center for the Prevention and Treatment
of Child Abuse and Neglect
Denver, Colorado

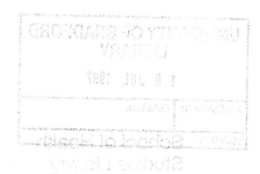

W. B. SAUNDERS COMPANY

Harcourt Brace Jovanovich, Inc.

Philadelphia   London   Toronto   Montreal   Sydney   Tokyo

W. B. SAUNDERS COMPANY
Harcourt Brace Jovanovich, Inc.

The Curtis Center
Independence Square West
Philadelphia, Pennsylvania 19106

Library of Congress Cataloging in Publication

Krugman, Richard D.
    Review of pediatrics / Richard D. Krugman.—4th ed.
        p. cm.
    Companion v. to Nelson textbook of pediatrics. 14th ed.
    ISBN 0-7216-3529-6
    1. Pediatrics—Examinations, questions, etc.   I. Nelson textbook of pediatrics.
    II. Title.
    [DNLM: 1. Pediatrics—examination questions.   WS 18 K94r]
RJ48.2.K78   1992   618.92′00076—dc20
DNLM/DLC   91-46791

REVIEW OF PEDIATRICS   ISBN   0-7216-3529-6

Printed in Mexico

Last digit is the print number: 9   8   7   6   5   4   3   2   1

This book is dedicated first to

my wife **MARY**

and to

(a) SCOTT
(b) JOSHUA
(c) TODD
(d) JORDAN

*All of the above have provided the proper perspective
for the pediatrician writing this book.*

*And also to Henry Kempe, Henry Silver, and Fred Battaglia,
all of whom have provided me an academic environment
in which I could thrive.*

Preface

Before plunging into the sea of multiple choice questions ahead, it would be wise to understand the philosophy underlying this book.

First, it is meant to be a companion to the *Nelson Textbook of Pediatrics,* fourteenth edition. When I was in the third grade, we had soft-cover "think and do books" that were handed out with our readers. (Bartholomew had how many hats? *a* 498 *b* 499 *c* 500 *d* other.) The purpose was to see if we had learned something about what we had read. It was *not* that we had to get 75% right or repeat the third grade. The distinction is important. Many review books prepare the reader specifically for exams and have "exam type" questions. These questions give multiple combination-type answers (choose "a" if 1 and 3 are correct, "b" if 2 and 5, etc.) I have avoided these because I am not sure whether questions worded in complex ways measure one's knowledge of pediatrics or one's ability to decipher instructions. Many of the questions you find in this book will tell you that four out of five answers are correct and ask you to choose the one that is incorrect. My hope is that this type of question will reinforce what you have already read once in the textbook. Past experience of hundreds of my students and residents is that this book *will* prepare you for exams—NBME PART II, ABP, and others.

Second, it should be noted that pediatrics is a heterogeneous field. Many approaches to the same problem exist, and indeed there is literature to support practically any point of view. If, as you go through this book, you are outraged at an answer or explanation that you believe is wrong, let me know. Many individuals did so after the first edition; few after the second, and fewer still after the third. Either I'm improving, or you're still not reading this preface.

Finally, it is important to remember that cognitive knowledge alone is not sufficient to care for children. Interpersonal skills, technical skills, and clinical judgment all are critical components of one's competence to practice pediatrics.

R.D.K.

Acknowledgments

Thanks to Mary Roth for typing and putting together this edition and my family and colleagues for giving me the time to do it.

Contents

1

The Field of Pediatrics

If you think about how textbooks are used, it is unlikely that the majority of people who buy or borrow a volume the size of the *Nelson Textbook of Pediatrics* read it cover to cover. Apart from the authors, the copy editors, a few compulsive third-year students, and myself, I suppose most readers are looking for a particular chapter or section so they can get a better handle on a patient they have just seen, or find a key reference or two so they can have something to say on morning rounds.

It is my guess then, that only a minority of you have read the opening chapter in the textbook. That's too bad, because there is more to pediatrics than the diseases of the heart, liver, and lungs, and "The Field of Pediatrics" gives an important perspective on this work. It traces the development of a specialty (as the next chapter is to trace the development of a child) and provides important insights into the significant contributions pediatrics has made to the health and well-being of children. The following questions will highlight major developments in the history of pediatrics, and look at some of the trends in the changing complexion of pediatric health care delivery in the 1980s.

1. Factors known to impact on the health problems of children include each of the following EXCEPT

   (a) ecology of infectious agents
   (b) climate and geography
   (c) astrologic influences
   (d) agricultural resources and practices
   (e) educational, economic, and sociocultural considerations

2. Each of the following statements concerning infant mortality is true EXCEPT

   (a) Approximately 20% of children born in the late 19th century in the United States could be expected to die during the first year of life
   (b) In 1925, the infant mortality rate in the United States was approximately 75 per 1000 live births
   (c) In 1988 the infant mortality rate in the United States was approximately 9.9 per 1000 live births
   (d) The majority of infant deaths in the United States in 1983 occurred during the first 28 days of life
   (e) Over the past 50 years, the mortality rate has decreased more markedly in infants up to 1 month of age than in the 1- to 11-month age group

3. Which of the following statements is false?

   (a) More children lived in single-parent families than two-parent families in 1986
   (b) Most children in single-parent families live with their mother
   (c) Most mothers work at least part time out of the house
   (d) In 1986, more than 20% of children under 5 years of age participated in day-care

4. Which of the following statements is true?

   (a) Between 1980 and 1987 the birthrate in the United States continued to decline
   (b) The adolescent population has continued to rise between 1980 and 1987
   (c) The number of children in the population is decreasing annually
   (d) Approximately half of office visits for children (<20 years) were to pediatricians

5. Which one of the following statements is false?

   (a) Homicide and suicide account for 25% of deaths in the 15- to 24-year-old age group
   (b) Motor vehicle accidents claim more children between 1 and 14 years of age than malignant neoplasms

(c) Homicide is a greater cause of death among 1- to 4-year-olds than meningitis

(d) As children get older, the overall mortality rate falls from a maximum in the first year of life to a minimum between 15 and 24 years of age

6. Which is true about the present costs of health care?

(a) Increased technology has made care more efficient and less costly

(b) Government insurance that reimburses physicians on a fee-for-service basis is the best hope for cost-containment in the next decade

(c) DRGs reimburse hospitals on the basis of diagnosis rather than actual costs

(d) Peer review has reduced costs to hospitals

7. The future of children at the hands of practitioners of pediatrics will best be served if

(a) the student or practitioner learns all the material in the textbook

(b) the student or practitioner learns all the material in the textbook and reads the current literature

(c) the student or practitioner learns to know the limits of his or her knowledge and recognizes when to call for help

(d) the trend toward subspecialization continues

2

Ethical and Cultural Issues in Pediatrics

It is refreshing to see this additional chapter in this edition of the Textbook. The increasing attention given to ethical and cultural issues in pediatrics parallels clinical practice throughout the United States and the world. With the extraordinary technologic developments in perinatal medicine, intrauterine (fetal) medicine and surgery, our recognition of the "rights" of children as well as their abuse, and an increased skepticism by society that the physician knows what is best for people, it is a rare week that goes by without some dilemma confronting us. Happily, a body of knowledge has begun to emerge which is synthesized in this chapter.

Just as "good ethics start with good facts" (a quote I learned from Norm Fost who wrote the section on ethics in Chapter 2), good practice begins with an appreciation of the cultural influences on our own and our patients' perspective on health, illness and its treatment. The answers to these questions will not be as factually based as those in later chapters, but the principles are very important to any student or practitioner.

QUESTIONS 1–5

Match the ethical principle (a–f) to the example given in the questions below.

1. _____ A physician obtains a court order to permit an appendectomy on a child over the religious objections of the parents
2. _____ Disclosure of biopsy result of a malignant tumor is withheld because no cure exists
3. _____ A 3-year-old is asked to consent to chemotherapy
4. _____ A physician is told by an adolescent that he is sexually involved with his 9-year-old sister
5. _____ A physician does not report suspected abuse because he feels the family will be harmed

   (a) Autonomy
   (b) Competence
   (c) Paternalism
   (d) Truth telling
   (e) Confidentiality
   (f) Conflict of interest

6. The "Baby Doe" dilemma refers to the legal issues surrounding
   (a) The prosecution of mothers giving birth at home and leaving their infants to die in trash dumpsters
   (b) The provision of blood transfusion in utero to erythroblastotic fetuses of a Jehovah's Witnesses mother
   (c) The withholding of medically beneficial treatment from infants with developmental disabilities
   (d) The placing of abandoned HIV-infected infants in foster homes

7. Each of the following is a characteristic of an "ideal ethical observer" in pediatric practice EXCEPT
   (a) consistency
   (b) omniscience
   (c) omnipercipience
   (d) disinterest and dispassion
   (e) an individual approach

8. Which of the following screening procedures has been most ethically sound from the perspective of newborns?
   (a) HIV (AIDS)
   (b) Phenylketonuria (PKU)

(c) Cystic fibrosis
(d) Fetal monitoring

9. Children are least protected in which of the following situations?

  (a) Therapeutic research with informed consent
  (b) Nontherapeutic research with informed consent
  (c) Innovative therapy with informed consent
  (d) All are equally dangerous

10. Which of the following is likely to be the least difficult ethical clinical situation in the early 1990s of those listed?

  (a) Conflict arising from pregnant woman using cocaine or other illicit drugs
  (b) Use of anencephalic infants for organ donations
  (c) Provision of contraceptive and sexually transmitted disease (STD) counseling
  (d) Delivery of a distressed 26-week premature infant by cesarian section to a mother with placenta previa refusing to consent to an operation

11. Each of the following has been positively correlated with acculturation EXCEPT

  (a) Residence in an ethnic enclave
  (b) Level and location of formal education
  (c) Length of time in host country
  (d) Ease in speaking the host language

12. Compliance with traditional medical approaches is more likely to occur if

  (a) the physician always makes eye contact when giving instructions
  (b) the physician uses a family friend as an interpreter
  (c) medication is prescribed with culturally acceptable foods
  (d) fold practices are recognized as being "Old World" and should be abandoned

QUESTIONS 13–15

Match the folk illness with its remedy.

13. _____ Empacho
14. _____ Mal (de) ojo
15. _____ Caida de mollera

  (a) rehydration
  (b) herbal teas, dietary restriction
  (c) benediction

3

Growth and Development

This chapter of the textbook is a tour through the diverse realm of developmental pediatrics. It walks us through physical, emotional, and intellectual development, and through broad issues related to adolescence, the retarded and the learning-disabled child, as well as the abused child. The basics of history-taking and physical examination are included, as is an approach to ethical issues.

The complex and diverse subject matter does not easily lend itself to questions regarding management, so the emphasis in this chapter will be on questions that call for factual information. Many will be exclusionary (i.e., each of the following is true EXCEPT). Hopefully, these will serve as a refresher so you can at least learn four true statements—instead of my trying to dream up four not-so-absurd-and-slightly-tricky alternatives to the one true answer.

At any rate, this chapter bears your attention. For one thing, the study of growth and development is what sets pediatrics apart from other specialties. Secondly, the focus of pediatrics in the coming decade will be turned more toward these areas than ever before. Many parents now are more interested in knowing how to rear a "normal child" than were their parents, who were reassured to know simply that their baby was not abnormal.

1. Which of the following statements regarding growth and development is true?

   (a) Physical growth and development proceed at a constant rate from birth to adolescence
   (b) The intellectual development of infants is best measured through neurologic and behavioral milestones
   (c) Emotional growth and development begin with the infant's ability to verbalize needs
   (d) Growth and development are guided principally by environmental forces

2. In a skewed population, which value is most representative of that population?

   (a) Average
   (b) Norm
   (c) Median
   (d) Mode

QUESTIONS 3–5

You are a student about to see your first pediatric patient in a well-baby clinic. Before going into the examining room, you notice that the growth chart of the 2-week-old infant you are about to see indicates that he is below the third percentile for weight and length and between the third and tenth percentiles for head circumference.

3. Which one of the following is most appropriate?

   (a) Assume that this is a case of failure to thrive and look for your supervisor
   (b) Proceed to the room to take a history and perform a physical examination
   (c) Call the laboratory for the results of the routine newborn thyroid screening test
   (d) Ask the nurse to weigh and measure the baby again

4. When you finally see the child and begin to take a history, which one of the following questions is most important to your management?

   (a) What are the heights and weights of the parents and grandparents?

(b) Is there a family history of thyroid disease, particularly in the mother?
(c) What was the baby's birth weight and length?
(d) What is the baby's nutritional intake?
(e) Is there a family history of hydrocephalus?

5. Which one of the following is the next-most-important question?
   (a) What was the infant's gestational age at birth?
   (b) Did the pregnancy go well?
   (c) How is the mother feeling?
   (d) Are there siblings who were under the third percentile for length and weight at this age?
   (e) Does the infant have any neurologic defects?

---

6. Each of the following statements is true EXCEPT

   (a) Intrauterine development consists of two phases—embryonic and fetal
   (b) Organogenesis is a second-trimester phenomenon
   (c) The embryonic period lasts 8 to 12 weeks
   (d) The fetus is viable at 24 to 26 weeks
   (e) The third trimester is one of growth rather than differentiation

7. Which one of the following has the least adverse effect on fetal growth and development?

   (a) Chromosomal abnormality
   (b) Viral and bacterial infection
   (c) Radiation, chemical, or other injury
   (d) Acute nutritional disturbance in a previously well-nourished mother
   (e) Chronic malnutrition in the mother

8. Each statement below is correct about fetal growth and development EXCEPT

   (a) Respiratory movements do not occur until birth
   (b) Swallowing movements commence as early as 14 weeks' gestation
   (c) Hemoglobin is primarily fetal
   (d) The grasp reflex is present at 17 weeks
   (e) Bile and meconium are present by 16 weeks

9. Each of the following is normal in a newborn infant EXCEPT

   (a) closure of the ductus venosus
   (b) closure of the ductus arteriosus
   (c) closure of the umbilical artery
   (d) higher proportion of extracellular water than in later life
   (e) greater ability to concentrate urine than in later life

10. A complete blood count in a normal, well newborn infant (24 hours old) is likely to have which of the following, relative to that of a normal, well 24-month-old child?

    (a) Higher hemoglobin, higher leukocyte count
    (b) Higher hemoglobin, lower leukocyte count
    (c) Lower hemoglobin, higher leukocyte count
    (d) Lower hemoglobin, lower leukocyte count

11. Visual fixation by newborn infants is associated with which Prechtl behavioral state?

    (a) Drowsy
    (b) Quiet, alert
    (c) Awake, active
    (d) Crying

12. Which one of the following tests best demonstrates that the newborn infant is capable of complex behavior?

    (a) Apgar score
    (b) Brazelton's Neonatal Behavioral Assessment Scale
    (c) Denver Developmental Screening Test
    (d) Wechsler Intelligence Scale for Children

13. Newborns have been shown to be able to do which of the following?

    (a) Preferentially respond to figures resembling a human face
    (b) Preferentially respond to higher-pitched rather than lower-pitched voices
    (c) Preferentially respond to the sound of their mother's voice
    (d) Recognize the mother's odor
    (e) All of the above
    (f) None of the above

14. Each of the following statements about the growth and development of prematurely born infants is true EXCEPT

 (a) A 1000- to 1500-gram infant is generally atonic with weak grasp, weak vocalizations, and a poor suck
 (b) A 2000-gram infant has a complete Moro response
 (c) Premature infants are indistinguishable from term infants developmentally once term gestational age is attained
 (d) Impaired motor and intellectual function are more common in prematurely born infants than their term counterparts
 (e) Premature infant-parental bonding and attachment may be more problematic than in term infants

QUESTIONS 15–24

For each of the following parental concerns, mark "N" if the finding is normal, or "C" if you would be concerned.

15. _____ My 1-week-old baby is the same weight now as when he was born
16. _____ My 11-month-old infant has no teeth
17. _____ The "soft spot" on my baby's head is larger now at 2 months than it was last month
18. _____ My 10-week-old infant isn't smiling when I smile at him
19. _____ My 4-month-old does not roll over from back to front yet
20. _____ My 8-month-old won't go to the baby sitter anymore without crying
21. _____ My 18-month-old isn't eating as well as before
22. _____ My 4-year-old is constantly touching his penis
23. _____ My 18-month-old doesn't talk in a way that anyone would recognize
24. _____ My 2½-year-old isn't toilet-trained

25. A mother brings her 6½-month-old boy to you for a "sick" visit. You saw the child 2 weeks earlier for health maintenance, including a DTP injection, and everything was fine. The mother's complaint is that the baby is waking up every night and is fussy during the day, especially when she leaves him. History is otherwise normal, and physical examination reveals no problems. Which one of the following is most appropriate?

 (a) Urinalysis and complete blood count to rule out urinary tract infection
 (b) Clear fluid diet for 24 hours in case the infant has mild gastroenteritis or is recting to something in the mother's breast milk
 (c) Reassure the mother that the behavior is normal and will pass in time
 (d) Reassure the mother that the behavior will pass because it is a reaction to the DTP shot

26. Which are the first *permanent* teeth to erupt?

 (a) Central incisors
 (b) Lateral incisors
 (c) Bicuspids
 (d) First molars (6-year molars)

27. The head is proportionately much larger than the rest of the body in

 (a) a 1-year-old as compared with a 6-year-old
 (b) a 6-year-old as compared with a 3-year-old
 (c) an adolescent as compared with a newborn
 (d) an adolescent as compared with an adult

28. The second year of life is characterized by each of the following EXCEPT

 (a) decreased appetite
 (b) deceleration of rate of weight gain
 (c) head circumference growing approximately ⅙ of first-year growth
 (d) eruption of 8 teeth
 (e) independent, nonimitative behavior

29. A 5-year-old boy is brought to you by his mother who is concerned because the child is "never well." Further history reveals that he has had one acute illness every 4 to 6 weeks since fall. Growth and development have been normal, and physical examination is negative except for large tonsils. Which of the following would you do?

 (a) Obtain a throat culture and reassure the mother that this number of acute illnesses is normal for a 5-year-old child starting school

(b) Order a laboratory evaluation including complete blood count, urinalysis, erythrocyte sedimentation rate, throat culture, and immunoglobulins
(c) Begin monthly injections of immune serum globulin, 0.66 ml/kg
(d) Administer prophylactic penicillin, 250 mg 2 times daily for 10 days
(e) Consider tonsillectomy and adenoidectomy

30. Each of the following is a significant medical problem in adolescents EXCEPT

(a) accidents
(b) acne
(c) suicide
(d) appendicitis and Meckel diverticulum
(e) nutritional problems (overnutrition/undernutrition)

QUESTIONS 31–35

For each set of physical findings listed below, select the appropriate Tanner sexual maturity rating (SMR 1 to 5).

31. _____ Preadolescent penis and testes with no pubic hair
32. _____ Sparse, lightly pigmented pubic hair, breast and papilla elevated
33. _____ Mature beasts, adult feminine triangle of pubic hair
34. _____ Coarse, curly pubic hair with aerola and papilla forming a secondary mound
35. _____ Slight enlargement of penis and scrotum with scanty pubic hair

36. The most rapid increase in height in girls is found in which Tanner SMR stage?

(a) 1
(b) 2
(c) 3
(d) 4
(e) 5

37. The most rapid increase in height in boys is found in which Tanner SMR stage?

(a) 1
(b) 2
(c) 3
(d) 4
(e) 5

38. Which one of the following correlates better with chronologic age than with the Tanner SMR stage?

(a) Serum alkaline phosphatase
(b) Hemoglobin concentration
(c) School performance (academic)
(d) Nutritional (caloric) requirements

39. Normal psychologic growth during adolescence requires each of the following EXCEPT

(a) emotional separation from the family
(b) physical separation from the family
(c) development of appropriate sexuality
(d) commitment to the future (e.g., vocation)
(e) achieving ego identity

40. Adolescent patients with asthma, diabetes, or other illnesses comply poorly with their treatments and tend to relapse often because of which of the following?

(a) An inability to find time in busy academic and extracurricular schedules to follow prescribed course
(b) A feeling that all adults, including the physican prescribing drugs, are "the enemy"
(c) A feeing that they do not want to be "hooked" on any drugs
(d) A feeling of immortality with no thought of the future consequences of their actions
(e) A general moodiness and recalcitrance

41. Early adolescents (10 to 13 years) exhibit each of the following psychosocial characterisics EXCEPT

(a) independence from family initiated
(b) heterosexual relationships
(c) conformity to peer groups
(d) sex differences in certain educational competencies
(e) beginning of "moral devleopment"

42. Domain-specific knowledge is a feature of

(a) Kohlberg's theory
(b) Piagetian theory
(c) Freudian theory
(d) Erickson's theory

43. Which statement is true?

(a) Ossification of the clavicles is rarely apparent at birth

(b) Fusion of the humeral capitellum will precede menarche by 1 year in girls

(c) Distal femoral and proximal tibial epiphyses are usually not ossified until 6 months of age

(d) Ossification charts available to assess adolescent bone age are more precise for boys than girls

44. Which statement is true concerning sulfonamide metabolism?

(a) Newborn drug metabolism is similar to older childhood

(b) Androgen effect on cytochrome P450 system impairs metabolism in male adolescents

(c) Acetylation is an autosomal recessive trait

(d) Hyperactive children with attention deficit disorder metabolize the drug differently

45. An 18-month-old child fails two parts of the Denver Developmental Screening Test (DDST): one in gross motor, one in fine motor. Which of the following is the appropriate interpretation?

(a) Normal

(b) Questionable—repeat test in 2 to 3 months

(c) Questionable—refer patient for further studies

(d) Abnormal—repeat test in 2 to 3 months

(e) Abnormal—refer patient for further studies

46. The DDST is best described as which one of the following?

(a) A behavioral assessment scale

(b) An intelligence test for preschool children and infants

(c) A developmental test to diagnose retardation

(d) A screening test to identify children needing further evaluation

QUESTIONS 47–50

Match the conceptual model or state of child development with its author/proponent.

47. _____ Psychoanalytic

48. _____ Cognitive model

49. _____ Separation-individuation

50. _____ Interaction of person and society

(a) Mahler

(b) Freud

(c) Erickson

(d) Piaget

(e) Brazelton

51. Chess and Thomas have described each of the following EXCEPT

(a) Nine characteristics that categorize temperamental styles of children

(b) "Difficult" children who have irregular biologic rhythms

(c) "Easy" children who are biologically predictable

(d) "Slow-to-warm" children who are shy, mildly negative, and somewhat intense

(e) Future behavioral problems most likely in the "slow-to-warm" group

52. What advice would you give to parents asking about the optimal spacing between children?

(a) 12 to 18 months

(b) 18 to 24 months

(c) 24 to 36 months

(d) More than 36 months

(e) Other

53. Vacillation between dependence and autonomy with respect to feelings toward parents is a characteristic behavior of which of the following age groups?

(a) Newborns and school age (5 to 12 years)

(b) Toddlers (18 to 30 months) and adolescents

(c) Kindergarten and college age

(d) Toddlers and school age

(e) 6-month-olds and toddlers

54. Important factors in promoting approved behavior in children include each of the following EXCEPT

(a) appropriate timing of punishment

(b) appropriate intensity of punishment

(c) consistency of approach

(d) parents' need for emotional outlet

(e) reinforcement of correct behavior

55. Which of the following is LEAST likely to cause poor school performance in a 7-year-old child?

(a) Progressive demyelinating disease
(b) Myopia
(c) Hearing deficit resulting from serous otitis media
(d) Emotional problems in the child's family
(e) Inadequate teaching in school

56. Which statistic regarding adolescent sexual behavior in the United States, as measured by percent having sexual intercourse, is correct?

(a) 68% of 13-year-old boys
(b) 10% of 15-year-old boys
(c) 20% of 19-year-old girls
(d) 80% of 19-year-old boys

57. Anxiety and depression are normal aspects of adolescent development. Appropriate methods of dealing with these problems include all of the following EXCEPT

(a) early emancipation of the adolescent by the parent
(b) involvement in extracurricular activities
(c) development of academic pursuits
(d) encouragement of a sense of humor in the adolescent
(e) encouragement of nonparental support mechanisms (e.g., group discussions)

58. Late adolescence is characterized by

(a) intimacy
(b) identity
(c) moral development
(d) depression

59. Each of the following is appropriate for a 4- to 5-year-old-child EXCEPT

(a) skips
(b) imitates a 5-cube "gate"
(c) remembers 6 forward and 5 reverse digits
(d) hops on one foot
(e) dresses and undresses self

60. An infant begins to mimic sounds at the same age it

(a) responds to its own name
(b) mimics pitch variations
(c) recognizes words like "mama" and "daddy"
(d) stops activity in response to "no"

QUESTIONS 61–62

A grandmother calls because she is concerned about her 2½-year-old grandson who has been fussy, crying a lot, difficult to get to sleep, and wetting the bed. His appetite has decreased markedly. He has no fever or other symptoms of illness. The child's parents are away on vacation.

61. Which of the following is the most likely cause of the child's symptoms?

(a) Allergic dermatitis
(b) Subclinical viral infection
(c) Urinary tract infection
(d) Small subdural hematoma secondary to trauma
(e) The parents' absence

62. When the parents return from vacation, their son is most likely to greet them with

(a) excitement
(b) indifference
(c) anger
(d) fear

QUESTIONS 63–64

63. Children at 5 to 6 years of age most often react to the death of a parent with

(a) guilt
(b) anxiety
(c) denial
(d) depression

64. Such children should be

(a) discouraged from attending the funeral
(b) encouraged to participate in the funeral
(c) given time alone to work through their feelings
(d) kept out of school, sports, and other activities for a prolonged period

65. "Permanency planning" refers to

(a) institutionalization of developmentally handicapped children
(b) limitation on moves by military families

(c) the use of adoptive placements or permanent foster care for abused children

(d) development of educational plans for developmentally handicapped children

66. Each of the following may be sequelae of parental divorce and separation EXCEPT

(a) Grief acutely

(b) Subsequent (5 years later) intense unhappiness

(c) Good adjustment after 10 years in 60 to 70% of children

(d) Academic and social problems after 10 years in 40% of children

(e) Problems with intimacy as an adult in many cases

67. Each of the following statements about television viewing by children is true EXCEPT

(a) Television viewing may enhance cognitive development

(b) Violent shows increase aggressive behavior in children

(c) Children in the United States watch less than 10 hours weekly

(d) Television viewing puts children in a passive observer role

68. School-age children generally react to chronic stress by any of the following mechanisms EXCEPT

(a) temper tantrums

(b) phobias

(c) impaired interpersonal relationships

(d) impaired school performance

(e) regressive behavior

69. Which one of the following statements regarding post-traumatic psychiatric disorders in children is true?

(a) Psychiatric disorders are as common in brain-injured children as they are in children without brain injury

(b) There is a typical pattern of psychiatric symptoms that follows injury, intoxication, or infection of the brain

(c) There is a significantly greater incidence of psychiatric disease in epileptic children as compared with children who do not have epilepsy

(d) More boys than girls develop post-traumatic psychiatric disorders

70. Which one of the following is LEAST typical of conversion reactions?

(a) Sudden onset

(b) Intra-abdominal or cardiac target organs

(c) A precipitating event

(d) No objective findings on physical examination

(e) Suggestive family history

71. Each of the following statements about psycho-physiologic disorders is true EXCEPT

(a) Onset is usually insidious

(b) Functional abnormalities of autonomic nervous system lead to organic changes

(c) Eczema, asthma, and colitis are examples of diseases with a psychosomatic component

(d) Children having such disorders are generally relaxed and outgoing, rarely obsessive-compulsive

72. Characteristics of anorexia nervosa include all of the following EXCEPT

(a) voluntary starvation, often beginning as a diet

(b) obsessive-compulsive behavior pattern prior to appearance of symptoms

(c) more common in girls than in boys

(d) depressed level of activity

(e) hospitalization required in moderate to severe cases

73. Pica is associated with each of the following EXCEPT

(a) iron deficiency anemia

(b) lead intoxication

(c) obesity

(d) moderate to severe mental retardation

(e) family disorganization and poor supervision

74. Which one of the following statements regarding enuresis in children is true?

(a) Diurnal enuresis in 5-year-old children is common and should be treated with reassurance only

(b) Diurnal enuresis in 5-year-old children is uncommon and should be evaluated and treated with imipramine (Tofranil)

(c) Nocturnal enuresis occurs in approximately 7% of normal 5-year-old boys

(d) Enuresis is more common in girls than boys

(e) Enuresis is effectively treated with electronic conditioning devices

75. Which of the following statements about encopresis and its treatment is true?

(a) The age at which bowel training is complete is the same at which day and night bladder control is achieved

(b) Encopresis in school-aged children should be viewed as a symptom of a serious disturbance and evaluated

(c) Encopresis is seen only slightly less commonly than enuresis in pediatric practice

(d) Chronic use of enemas and laxatives is to be encouraged to prevent encopresis

76. Sleep disturbances would be normal in which of the following children?

(a) A 6- to 9-month-old infant

(b) A 2- to 3-year-old with nightmares

(c) A 5-year-old just starting school

(d) An 8-year-old whose parents are separated

(e) All of these

77. Head banging, hair twirling, rocking, thumb sucking, teeth grinding, and nail biting, are all

(a) habit disorders that probably relieve tension

(b) easy to cure in children

(c) evidence of insecurity in the majority of children and of poor parenting by their parents

(d) tics

78. Each of the following statements about masturbation is true EXCEPT

(a) It is nearly universal among children and adolescents

(b) It is, if not carried to an extreme, normal at any age

(c) It permits the adolescent to explore newly discovered sexual capacities

(d) It should be ignored by parents in all cases since discussion will reinforce the behavior

79. Which of the following statements about suicide is true?

(a) Most suicidal children are psychotic (generally autistic)

(b) The suicide attempt is not sudden—most children are depressed for a month or more prior to the event

(c) Adolescent boys and girls are equally susceptible

(d) Most suicidal children have lower than average IQ

(e) With newer psychiatric techniques, hospitalization is rarely necessary

80. The best treatment for breath holding as a part of temper tantrums in children 2 to 3 years old is

(a) spanking

(b) mouth-to-mouth resuscitation

(c) ignoring the behavior and leaving the room

(d) prophylactic anticonvulsant medication and then ignoring the episodes

(e) making sure that the child never gets angry

81. Each of the following statements about attention deficit hyperactivity disorder (ADHD) is true EXCEPT

(a) The prevalence is 1.5 to 4.0% of school-aged children

(b) Boys are only slightly more often affected than girls

(c) Affected children are not really more active; rather, they are less purposeful and more fidgety

(d) There is no clear-cut cause

(e) Diagnosis before school age (5 to 6 years) is difficult, since many 2- to 4-year-olds who are very active do not become "hyperactive"

82. Which of the following is the ideal setting to evaluate ADHD?

(a) The child's classroom or home

(b) The pediatrician's office

(c) The psychologist's office

(d) A developmental evaluation center

83. Treatment of children with ADHD should be *primarily* directed toward

(a) structuring the child's environment

(b) helping the parents cope

(c) beginning a drug regimen

(d) looking for a better school

(e) reassuring parents and school personnel that the symptoms will pass with time

84. Side effects of drug therapy (dextroamphetamine or methylphenidate) for hyperactivity include each of the following EXCEPT

(a) anorexia

(b) insomnia

(c) growth suppression

(d) tachycardia

(e) dependence (addiction)

85. Which of the following is evidence of aberrant behavior?

(a) A 4-year-old boy and girl undressing and touching each other's genitalia

(b) A 4½-year-old boy dressing up in his mother's clothes

(c) Secretive cross-dressing in a 7-year-old boy

(d) Cross-dressing in an 11-year-old girl

86. Each of the following statements concerning autism is true EXCEPT

(a) The child is withdrawn and avoids human contact

(b) There are many compulsive routines

(c) The exact cause is unknown, but it is most likely a reaction to an adverse parental environment

(d) Head banging, rocking, and self-mutilation are common

(e) therapeutic efforts are generally fruitless

87. Each of the following statements is true EXCEPT

(a) Homosexual orientation is not fixed until middle to late adolescence

(b) Effeminacy in boys may be benign if not accompanied by cross-dressing

(c) Voyeurism is common in preschool children

(d) Exhibitionism is benign at all ages, and the most common reported "deviancy"

QUESTIONS 88–89

A mother brings a 3-week-old baby to the emergency room at 1:00 AM with a chief complaint of rash and irritability. On examination (less than compulsive at that hour) you find a peacefully sleeping baby and no rash.

88. Appropriate action on your part would be to

(a) obtain more history

(b) order a complete blood count and urinalysis

(c) reassure the mother that the rash has disappeared and tell her to come back if it returns

(d) make an appointment for her at the dermatology clinic and lecture her about the proper use of an emergency room

(e) admit the baby for evaluation of sepsis

89. On further questioning you learn that the mother really came to the emergency room because the child's father had threatened her and the baby, and when the baby began crying, she felt like killing it. *Now* what do you do?

(a) Admit the baby immediately and notify the police and child protection team

(b) Reassure the mother that occasionally feeling like killing her child is not abnormal, although actually doing so would be, and send her home with an appointment to see a social worker in the morning

(c) Reassure the mother that her feelings are not abnormal, and ask her where she and the baby would feel most safe— the hospital, with a relative or friend, or elsewhere—and call the child protection team *before* she leaves

(d) Suggest she notify the police to protect her and the baby, and make an appointment for the local social services department to investigate the case in the morning

90. All of the following statements about child abuse and neglect in the United States are true EXCEPT

(a) Approximately 2% of the children in the United States are abused or neglected

(b) Premature infants are at greater risk than full-term infants

(c) Child abuse rarely occurs in upper socioeconomic groups

(d) 2000 to 4000 children die yearly; many more are severely affected
(e) The majority of delinquent children and runaway adolescents have been abused

91. Which of the following statements regarding child abuse is true?

(a) Most abusive parents are psychotic
(b) Abuse requires a parent with a specific motive, a child who has specific characteristics, and a crisis to precipitate the event
(c) Most abuse is premeditated
(d) The incidence of child abuse among military families is relatively low, since health care is generally readily available
(e) The treatment of abusive parents is generally unrewarding, and thus they should be prosecuted

92. Which statement is true about sexual abuse?

(a) The physical examination is usually diagnostic in prepubertal children
(b) Forensic studies ("rape exams") are rarely useful in prepubertal children and should be avoided
(c) The use of "anatomically correct" dolls is leading and traumatic to young children
(d) A positive chlamydia slide test is diagnostic of sexual abuse
(e) A child's statement about abuse is usually true and must be reported

93. Examples of developmental dysfunction in the school-aged child include all of the following EXCEPT

(a) hyperactivity syndrome
(b) visual-spatial disorganization
(c) temporal-sequential disorganization
(d) memory deficits
(e) language dysfunction

94. Each of the following is typical of reading problems EXCEPT

(a) Narrative dysfluency
(b) Poor decoding
(c) Delayed comprehension
(d) Incomplete recall
(e) Deficient summarization

95. Which of the following would be LEAST appropriate for dealing with a child with a learning disability who is failing in school?

(a) Repeating the year, since the material will be more familiar the second time
(b) Attention of classroom structure (e.g., changing from an "open" classroom to a conventional "closed" one)
(c) Modification of teacher behavior
(d) Modification of the curriculum
(e) Specialized remedial help

96. Which of the following is true about chronic illness in childhood?

(a) In contrast to adults, it is quite common for children to have chronic illness
(b) The percentage of children with chronic illness is falling as technology advances
(c) The burden of care for chronic illness is borne by society
(d) Most illnesses require a multidisciplinary approach

QUESTIONS 97–100

Match the diagnostic test (a–e) appropriate to assess the mentally retarded child in the case given.

97. _____ Enlarging head
98. _____ Acrodermatitis
99. _____ Abnormal genitalia
100. _____ Self-mutilation

(a) Uric acid (serum)
(b) Serum zinc
(c) Chromosomal karyotype
(d) CT scan or MRI
(e) EEG

4

Nutrition and Nutritional Disorders

A legislator I know visited a medical school 20 years ago to see how his state's tax dollars were being spent. Halfway through the day, he jumped to his feet and asked, "Who teaches nutrition here?" The Dean carefully explained that many departments taught nutrition. Biochemistry, physiology, internal medicine, surgery, pediatrics, and obstetrics all included lectures in nutrition, and there was even an elective in nutrition offered to first-year students.

"Not enough!" boomed the legislator. "Good nutrition is the basis of good health. How can you not give doctors the knowledge they need to take care of people? You should have a Department of Nutrition!"

My presumption is that most of you reading this book have *not* been to a school with a Department of Nutrition, and, in fact, that school *still* doesn't. As a result, many of you may have brushed over this chapter in the textbook. If you did, go back.

Nutrition is the driving force behind growth and development, and we already said at the beginning of the last chapter that growth and development are what set pediatrics apart from other specialties. So, as important as nutrition is in general, it is particularly crucial to understand basic concepts of nutrition for children. You should resist the temptation to skip ahead to inborn errors of metabolism or cardiology, and should pay attention to the sections on nutrition. They lead from basic discussions of water, proteins, calories, and the like to a guide to feeding techniques, and finally to a dissertation on vitamins and nutritional disorders. Unlike some of the questions in the previous chapters, intuition alone won't carry you through.

1. Which one of the following statements regarding the water requirements of infants is true?

   (a) Infants require much more water per 100-calorie intake than adults do
   (b) Infants' water requirements per kilogram of body weight are about the same as adults'
   (c) Requirements depend on variables such as renal solute load, dietary protein content, and body temperature
   (d) Water requirements are decreased in premature infants receiving phototherapy

2. The caloric need of infants is easily gauged by
   (a) adding calories used in basal metabolism, specific dynamic action, exercise, and growth
   (b) looking at growth pattern, sense of well-being, and satiety

   (c) calculating intake of protein, fat, and carbohydrate
   (d) measuring stool fat

3. Each of the following is an essential amino acid EXCEPT

   (a) threonine
   (b) glutamine
   (c) valine
   (d) lysine
   (e) tryptophan

QUESTIONS 4–8

For each ingested substrate, select the enzyme involved in its digestion (a–e).

4. _____ Medium-chain triglycerides   (a) Amylase
              (b) Pancreatic lipase
5. _____ Proteoses and peptones   (c) Disaccharidase

6. _____ Starch   (d) Phosphorylase
7. _____ Lactose   (e) Trypsin
8. _____ Maltose

9. Which of the following are synthesized in the human gastrointestinal tract?

   (a) Vitamins A, C, and E
   (b) Vitamins B_{12}, D, and K
   (c) Vitamin K, pantothenic acid, and biotin
   (d) Vitamins E and K and biotin
   (e) Vitamin K, riboflavin, and flavonoids

10. Each of the following trace elements is important in human metabolism EXCEPT

   (a) copper
   (b) zinc
   (c) iron
   (d) chromium
   (e) manganese

11. Sources of copper in the diet include each of the following EXCEPT

   (a) milk
   (b) liver
   (c) fish
   (d) nuts
   (e) legumes

12. A dietary source of the trace element chromium is

   (a) liver
   (b) oysters
   (c) yeast
   (d) eggs
   (e) meat

13. Instructions to mothers leaving the nursery with their normal full-term infants with regard to feeding should include which of the following?

   (a) Crying infants are hungry infants
   (b) Infants will set their own schedule, but in no case should more than 4 hours elapse between feedings
   (c) Disinterest in food may be a sign of illness
   (d) Adding cereal to the diet will cause the child to sleep through the night sooner
   (e) Juices should be given to newborns as an excellent source of vitamin C

QUESTIONS 14–22

For each of these statements, mark "A" if the statement is true of breast milk only, "B" if it is true of formula only, "C" if it is true of both, or "D" if it is true for neither.

14. _____ Contains approximately 20 calories per ounce
15. _____ Gatrointestinal allergy less common
16. _____ Free of bacterial contamination
17. _____ Contains secretory IgA antibodies
18. _____ Associated with increased mortality rates in lower socioeconomic groups
19. _____ Associated with decreased incidence of colic and eczema
20. _____ Associated with prolonged unconjugated hyperbilirubinemia
21. _____ Weight gain over first 2 weeks is greater
22. _____ Carbohydrate concentration is higher, whereas protein concentration is lower

23. The mother of a 1-week-old infant calls because she is concerned about her infant's bowel movements. She reports six to ten soft watery stools each day. Further questioning reveals that there is no fever, the infant is actively nursing, and there are 10 to 12 wet diapers daily. Which of the following statements is true?

   (a) If the infant is breast-fed, this is a worrisome history
   (b) The stool pattern is normal for a breast-fed infant
   (c) The stool pattern described is normal for formula-fed infants who are getting supplemental cereal
   (d) This history is suggestive of a milk-borne diarrheal epidemic in the hospital nursery

24. Three weeks later she calls back and says that the baby hasn't had a stool for 6 days. The baby is still nursing, is not fussy, and is otherwise well. Which statement is the proper course?

   (a) Schedule a flat plate X-ray of the abdomen
   (b) Suggest use of a suppository
   (c) Refer to a gastroenterologist for rectal biopsy
   (d) Provide reassurance and follow-up by telephone

QUESTIONS 25–33

For each of the following milk preparations, mark "A" if it is satisfactory for routine feeding of newborns only, "B" if it is satisfactory for older children only, "C" if satisfactory for both, or "D" if satisfactory for neither.

25. _____ Sweetened condensed milk
26. _____ Homogenized whole cow's milk
27. _____ Evaporated milk (diluted 1:1.5 with water)
28. _____ Goat's milk
29. _____ Soy-based formula
30. _____ Nondairy coffee lightener (e.g., Pream)
31. _____ 2% "low-fat" cow's milk
32. _____ Nonfat dry milk (reconstituted)
33. _____ Raw milk

---

34. Supplemental vitamin D is necessary in infants who are

    (a) breast-fed
    (b) fed commercial formulas (e.g., Similac, Enfamil)
    (c) given evaporated milk formulas
    (d) residents of the "sun belt"

35. The best source of iron for 3-month-old infants is

    (a) iron-fortified cereals
    (b) yellow vegetables
    (c) fruits
    (d) breast milk
    (e) 2% "low-fat" cow's milk

36. Each of the following may be a cause of loose stools in an infant EXCEPT

    (a) overfeeding
    (b) starvation
    (c) excessive sugar content of formula
    (d) ingestion of codeine analgesics by the mother of a breast-fed infant
    (e) viral infection

37. Nursing vegan mothers may have infants with which of the following problems?

    (a) Methylmalonic acidemia
    (b) Hyperlipidemia
    (c) Bulky stools
    (d) Increased gastrointestinal motility
    (e) Appendicitis

38. During the second year of life, which of the following statements is true?

    (a) Most children in the United States eat a well-balanced diet over a period of several days
    (b) Colic often occurs in the late afternoon or evening
    (c) Most children need to be fed by their parents to ensure an adequate nutritional intake
    (d) Vitamin deficiencies are common among American children
    (e) Caloric intake per unit body weight increases

39. Each of the following statements about kwashiorkor is true EXCEPT

    (a) It is a disease of the second child
    (b) Dermatitis is common
    (c) It is primarily a caloric malnutrition
    (d) The liver is enlarged with a fatty infiltration
    (e) Clinical signs include lack of growth, loss of muscle tissue, and edema

40. Each of the following is a feature of the pickwickian syndrome EXCEPT

    (a) marked obesity
    (b) somnolence
    (c) good response to oxygen therapy
    (d) cardiac enlargement
    (e) hypoventilation

41. Each of the following is associated with vitamin A deficiency EXCEPT

    (a) hyperkeratosis
    (b) increased vitamin D levels
    (c) celiac disease
    (d) chronic infectious diseases
    (e) chronic ingestion of mineral oil

42. Anorexia, alopecia, seborrhea, craniotabes, and increased intracranial pressure are all seen in

    (a) hypervitaminosis A
    (b) hypervitaminosis D
    (c) vitamin A deficiency
    (d) vitamin D deficiency

QUESTIONS 43–47

For each disorder, select the appropriate vitamin deficiency (a–f).

43. _____ Beriberi
44. _____ Scurvy
45. _____ Rickets
46. _____ Pellagra
47. _____ Night
    blindness

(a) Vitamin A
(b) Riboflavin
(c) Vitamin B_1
    (thiamine)
(d) Niacin
(e) Vitamin C
(f) Vitamin D

QUESTIONS 48–51

For each symptom of the deficiency disease, select the appropriate vitamin (a–f).

48. _____ Seizures, neuro-
    pathy
49. _____ Pseudoparalysis
50. _____ Craniotabes, en-
    larged costo-
    chondral junc-
    tions
51. _____ Dermatitis, diar-
    rhea dementia

(a) Vitamin A
(b) Vitamin B_1
    (thiamine)
(c) Niacin
(d) Vitamin B_6
    (pyridoxine)
(e) Vitamin C
(f) Vitamin D

52. Vitamin D does each of the following EX-CEPT

    (a) increases renal tubular reabsorption of phosphate
    (b) increases intestinal absorption of phosphate
    (c) increases intestinal absorption of calcium
    (d) increases reabsorption of calcium from bone

53. Vitamin E deficiency is associated with each of the following EXCEPT

    (a) thrombocytosis
    (b) decreased platelet adhesiveness
    (c) prematurity
    (d) malabsorption syndromes

QUESTIONS 54–57

A 3-week-old infant is brought to the emergency room in coma with retinal hemorrhages and severe pallor. He was born at home and was first seen by a physician at 10 days of age and placed on amoxicillin for otitis media. The day prior to admission his parents took him on a trip over a rough 4-wheel drive road in the mountains. Seizures began 8 hours later, and he steadily deteriorated over the next 16 hours. He oozes blood from all venipuncture sites.

54. Diagnostic tests should include all of the following EXCEPT

    (a) bleeding screen
    (b) skeletal survey
    (c) CT scan
    (d) trial of pyridoxine
    (e) lumbar puncture

55. Immediate therapy should include which one of the following?

    (a) Vitamin A
    (b) Vitamin B_6 (pyridoxine)
    (c) Vitamin C
    (d) Vitamin E
    (e) Vitamin K

56. This child's diagnosis is most likely

    (a) pyridoxine deficiency
    (b) severe scurvy
    (c) hemorrhagic disease of the newborn
    (d) child abuse
    (e) hypervitaminosis A

57. This death could have been prevented by which *one* of the following measures?

    (a) AquaMEPHYTON (vitamin K) at birth
    (b) Home-visitor services
    (c) Discontinuance of antibiotics
    (d) Proper use of infant seat

5
Preventive Pediatrics and Epidemiology

It is indicative of the place prevention has had in our health care system that this chapter is among the smallest in the textbook. Most of the chapter describes the sequence of preventive or health maintenance services prescribed for children in the United States, and in developing countries as well. The questions that follow reflect this emphasis.

QUESTIONS 1–5

For each of the following, mark "A" if the intervention is an example of primary prevention, "B" if secondary prevention, "C" if neither.

1. ____ Tetanus immunization
2. ____ Pap smears
3. ____ Water fluoridation
4. ____ Scoliosis screening
5. ____ Blood lead screening

---

6. Examples of preventive health services that are community responsibilities include each of the following EXCEPT

   (a) provision of safe milk
   (b) screening of children for hypertension with sphygmomanometry
   (c) reduction of air pollution
   (d) provision of adequate housing
   (e) fluoridation of water supplies

7. Each of the following has been effective in reducing the morbidity and mortality of childhood accidents EXCEPT

   (a) encouraging parental use of automobile seat restraints for children
   (b) "childproof" containers
   (c) flame-resistant fabrics
   (d) regulations to ensure safe spacing of crib rails
   (e) window guards for apartment buildings

8. The adolescent age group is least affected by which of the following?

   (a) Homicide
   (b) Poisoning
   (c) Suicide
   (d) Substance abuse
   (e) Pregnancy

9. Appropriate reasons for a pediatrician to have a prenatal visit with prospective parents include each of the following EXCEPT

   (a) to determine risk of genetic disease
   (b) to promote positive attitudes toward parenting
   (c) to discuss specific diseases that they need to be aware of in the first year
   (d) to establish a good relationship with them
   (e) to discuss the possibility of sibling rivalry

10. Which of the following statements is true concerning the frequency and timing of "well child" visits?

    (a) The first visit following discharge from the nursery should be at 3 to 4 weeks of age
    (b) Each visit during the first year is accompanied by an immunization
    (c) The timing and scheduling of visits should be individualized for each child
    (d) Once the child is school-aged, visits should occur at least once a year
    (e) Anticipatory guidance is primarily useful in the newborn period

11. Each of the following statements concerning education of parents by physicians is true EXCEPT

    (a) Most pediatricians spend little time doing it

(b) The effectiveness of parent education, as measured by behavioral change, is not proved

(c) Many pediatric training programs do not teach students how to educate parents

(d) Involvement of children or parents in education programs is less important now than it was before the availability of antibiotics

12. By 12 months of age all children should have had which of the following routinely?

(a) DTP $\times$ 3, TOPV $\times$ 2, MMR
(b) DTP $\times$ 3, TOPV $\times$ 2, smallpox vaccination
(c) DTP $\times$ 3, TOPV $\times$ 2
(d) DTP $\times$ 3, TOPV $\times$ 2, measles vaccine
(e) Td $\times$ 3, TOPV $\times$ 2

13. Which of the following is true of poliovirus vaccines licensed in the United States?

(a) IPV (Salk) is the preferred vaccine for routine use
(b) 95% of immunized children have antibody to all three types of polio after two doses of OPV
(c) OPV is safe for use in household contacts of immunocompromised children
(d) IPV requires more doses for protection of children than OPV
(e) Adult contacts of OPV immunized children *must* receive IPV before the children are immunized

QUESTIONS 14–17

Select the immunization (a–b) that each high-risk group of children (over age 2) should receive.

14. _____ Children with cystic fibrosis
15. _____ Children with sickle cell anemia
16. _____ Children with severe asthma
17. _____ Children with bronchopulmonary dysplasia

(a) Pneumococcal vaccine
(b) Influenza vaccine

18. The association of Reye syndrome and salicylate ingestion is an example of the use of which type of epidemiologic approach?

(a) Descriptive epidemiology
(b) Experimental epidemiology

(c) Prospective study
(d) Retrospective (case control) study

19. A retrospective epidemiologic study is most useful in assessing

(a) prevalence
(b) incidence
(c) relative risk
(d) absolute risk

QUESTIONS 20–21

For each pitfall in clinical study, select the probable type of bias (a–c) associated with it.

20. _____ A factor associated with the disease is also linked to the characteristic under study
21. _____ Control group differs in some inherent characteristic related to outcome that is different from the factor being studied

(a) Selection
(b) Observational
(c) Confounding

22. Developing countries have infant mortality rates in excess of 15%. The leading cause of death is

(a) infection (measles, pertussis, neonatal tetanus)
(b) diarrhea and malnutrition
(c) natural disasters (volcanoes, earthquakes, floods)
(d) war

23. Appropriate accident prevention advice for parents of children in their first year includes each of the following EXCEPT

(a) Keep crib sides up
(b) Use seat belts in the automobile
(c) Keep syrup of ipecac at home
(d) Do not leave the child alone in the bath
(e) Keep small objects (less than 2 cm) out of reach

24. Appropriate accident prevention advice for parents of preschoolers (2- to 4-year-olds) includes each of the following EXCEPT

(a) Keep screens or guards in windows
(b) Keep firearms locked away
(c) Teach two-wheel bicycle safety

(d) Use seat belts or other restraint in the automobile

(e) Keep knives and electrical equipment out of reach

25. Appropriate accident prevention advice for parents of elementary school children includes each of the following EXCEPT

(a) Use seat belts in the automobile
(b) Teach bicycle safety
(c) Keep firearms locked away
(d) Encourage swimming lessons
(e) Keep the child in an enclosed space if he or she is outdoors when no adult is present

QUESTIONS 26–40

For each of the following, mark "A" if the immunization is a live attenuated product, "B" if it is inactivated, "C" if a toxoid.

26. _____ Hepatitis B
27. _____ Rubella
28. _____ Diphtheria
29. _____ Pertussis
30. _____ Tetanus
31. _____ Salk polio
32. _____ Sabin polio
33. _____ Rabies
34. _____ Typhoid
35. _____ Mumps
36. _____ Measles
37. _____ Yellow fever
38. _____ Hib (HbCV)
39. _____ Cholera
40. _____ Meningococcal

6

General Considerations in the Care of the Sick Child

This chapter begins the long walk through the problems of sick children. The subject matter here is important. Fluids and electrolytes are the cornerstones of pediatric therapy, and unlike the adult situation ("15 and 5 with a bit of K"), there is little room for error in calculation.

If after reading this chapter and answering these questions you feel as though you are back in physiology, you will appreciate why basic science is important in medicine. Basic principles of pharmacology, CPR, treatment of shock, and burn therapy are also included.

It should be noted that there are numerous schemes for calculating fluid and electrolytes, and there is healthy debate over items such as the treatment of hypernatremic dehydration. However, the questions that follow relate specifically to the text, and not the general literature.

1. The clinical evaluation of a sick infant will vary LEAST from that of an adult patient in regard to which of the following?

   (a) The use of an "interpreter" (e.g., parent) as primary historian
   (b) The importance of understanding developmental variations
   (c) Laboratory data interpretation
   (d) The order and approach to a physical examination

2. Inspection, palpation, percussion and auscultation is the correct order for examination of each of the following EXCEPT

   (a) cardiac exam
   (b) abdominal exam
   (c) chest exam
   (d) examination of the head

3. Which of the following statements is true about well child (health supervision) visits?

   (a) The first visit should be at 2 weeks of age
   (b) The major purpose for each visit is to provide immunizations
   (c) Accident prevention and anticipatory guidance can be addressed in the context of the child's development
   (d) The Denver Developmental Screening test (DDST) should be performed on every visit

4. Which of the following is the most prevalent serious infectious febrile illness of infants under 36 months of age?

   (a) Pneumonia
   (b) Bacterial meningitis
   (c) Aseptic meningitis
   (d) Urinary tract infection

5. Total body water accounts for approximately what percentage of body weight in a 2-year-old child?

   (a) 90%
   (b) 75%
   (c) 60%
   (d) 50%
   (e) 33%

6. Extracellular fluid volume is larger than the intracellular fluid volume in which one of the following?

   (a) Fetus
   (b) Toddler
   (c) Adolescent
   (d) Adult

7. Which of the following is the largest component of the extracellular fluid?

   (a) Plasma water
   (b) Interstitial water
   (c) Gastrointestinal secretions
   (d) Cerebrospinal fluid

8. Obligatory water losses include each of the following EXCEPT

   (a) evaporation from lungs
   (b) evaporation from skin
   (c) urinary water necessary to excrete solute
   (d) stool water

9. Which one of the following occurs with decreased intravascular volume resulting from hemorrhage?

   (a) Thirst
   (b) Inhibition of antidiuretic hormone
   (c) Decreased plasma osmolality
   (d) Increased urinary flow
   (e) Increased evaporative water loss

10. The primary action of antidiuretic hormone is to

    (a) increase the effectiveness of the hypothalamus
    (b) increase the sensitivity of the supraoptic nuclei
    (c) increase the permeability of the renal collecting ducts to water
    (d) increase the tubular reabsorption of sodium

11. Which one of the following inhibits release of antidiuretic hormone?

    (a) Stress from burns, trauma, or surgery
    (b) Acute bacterial meningitis
    (c) Nicotine
    (d) Alcohol

12. The principal contributor to colloid osmotic pressure in the regulation of water movement across capillary walls is

    (a) sodium
    (b) chloride
    (c) free fatty acids
    (d) albumin

13. Dietary sodium is absorbed minimally in the

    (a) stomach
    (b) duodenum
    (c) jejunum
    (d) ileum

14. The sodium concentration is highest in which of the following transcellular fluids?

    (a) Saliva
    (b) Gastric juice
    (c Ileal fluid
    (d) Bile
    (e) Cerebrospinal fluid

15. Renal reabsorption of sodium occurs at each of the following EXCEPT

    (a) glomerulus
    (b) proximal convoluted tubule
    (c) loop of Henle
    (d) distal convoluted tubule
    (e) collecting duct

16. Aldosterone has which of the following physiologic effects?

    (a) Increases urinary excretion of sodium; decreases urinary excretion of potassium
    (b) Decreases urinary excretion of sodium; increases urinary excretion of potassium
    (c) Decreases systemic blood pressure
    (d) Acts on the proximal convoluted tubule with antidiuretic hormone to prevent water reabsorption
    (e) Increases both sodium and potassium excretion

17. Which pair of organs is most involved in potassium homeostasis?

    (a) Kidney, colon
    (b) Kidney, skin
    (c) Skin, colon
    (d) Muscle, kidney

18. Each of the following statements is true about the regulation of potassium EXCEPT

    (a) Potassium is freely filtered in the glomerulus
    (b) Mineralocorticoid action on the colon will increase the potassium content of the stool
    (c) For every 0.1 unit change in blood pH, plasma potassium moves 0.3 to 1.3 mEq in the opposite direction

(d) External losses of potassium results in a shift from intracellular to extracellular fluid

(e) Since most potassium is intracellular, there has to be a large increase in total body potassium to develop hyperkalemia

19. Calcium absorption from the gastrointestinal tract is increased by each of the following EXCEPT

(a) parathormone
(b) vitamin D
(c) pregnancy
(d) phytate, citrate, and oxalate
(e) decreased dietary intake of calcium

20. Which of the following is associated with hypercalcemia?

(a) Malabsorption
(b) Hypoparathyroidism
(c) Hyperphosphatemia
(d) Supravalvular aortic stenosis
(e) Infundibular pulmonic stenosis

21. Hypomagnesemia is associated with each of the following EXCEPT

(a) diuretic therapy
(b) maternal eclampsia therapy
(c) primary aldosteronism
(d) renal tubular acidosis
(e) malabsorption syndromes

22. Metabolic acidosis occurs with all of the following EXCEPT

(a) chronic renal insufficiency
(b) salicylism
(c) diarrhea
(d) Bartter syndrome
(e) starvation

23. Metabolic alkalosis occurs in which one of the following?

(a) Pyloric stenosis
(b) Methyl alcohol poisoning
(c) Ketogenic diet
(d) Hyperalimentation
(e) Excessive intake of ethyl alcohol

24. Respiratory alkalosis occurs in which one of the following?

(a) Pickwickian syndrome
(b) Hyperventilation syndrome

(c) Kyphoscoliosis
(d) Guillain-Barré syndrome

25. A 14-kg child has approximately what daily water requirement (maintenance)?

(a) 700 ml
(b) 1000 ml
(c) 1200 ml
(d) 1400 ml
(e) 2800 ml

26. Water should be replaced on a milliliter-for-milliliter basis in each of the following disease states EXCEPT

(a) anuria
(b) diuretic phase of acute tubular necrosis
(c) severe diarrhea
(d) vomiting in pyloric stenosis

27. Which of the following is NOT an expected laboratory finding in a child with moderate hyponatremic dehydration (10 to 12%)?

(a) Serum sodium 124 mEq/l
(b) Serum potassium 4.5 mEq/l
(c) Blood urea nitrogen 30 mg/dl
(d) Hematocrit 28%

28. The optimum initial therapy for severely dehydrated children is

(a) whole blood
(b) packed red blood cells
(c) plasma
(d) isotonic saline with glucose (5%)
(e) 10% dextrose in water

29. Oral rehydration solution is contraindicated in which of the following situations?

(a) Cholera
(b) Hyponatremic dehydration
(c) Diarrhea with severe gastric distension
(d) Isonatremic dehydration

30. The finding of a marked metabolic alkalosis with an acidic urine indicates which one of the following?

(a) Marked with sodium depletion
(b) Marked potassium depletion
(c) Hyperventilation
(d) Diabetes mellitus
(e) Laboratory error

31. Children with extensive burns lose fluids in proportion to

(a) their weight
(b) their surface area
(c) their percentage of surface area with second- or third-degree burns
(d) their metabolic rate
(e) their body temperature

32. The fluid and electrolyte management of acute salicylism should include each of the following EXCEPT

(a) rapid alkalinization with sodium bicarbonate (2 mEq/kg/hour)
(b) maintenance fluid over first 6 hours ($\sim$ 1200 ml/M^2/24 hours)
(c) large quantities of potassium both intravenously and orally
(d) maximum fluid (2 to 3 times maintenance)

33. Neonatal hypocalcemia and tetany is LEAST likely to occur in which of the following?

(a) Postmature, appropriate size-for-gestational-age (AGA) infants
(b) Premature AGA infants with respiratory distress
(c) Premature, small-for-gestational-age infants
(d) Infants of diabetic mothers
(e) Infants who had difficult deliveries

34. Each of the following statements is true about failure to thrive (FTT) EXCEPT

(a) Most cases have a nonorganic etiology
(b) Hospitalization is often diagnostic
(c) Extensive laboratory evaluation is indicated if history and physical exam are not helpful
(d) Factors associated with FTT include young parents, economic stress, and single parenthood
(e) Most children with FTT eventually develop normally with respect to physical growth

QUESTIONS 35–38

For each disease state, select the appropriate therapy (a–f).

35. _____ Hypokalemia
36. _____ Hyperkalemia
37. _____ Hypermagnesemia
38. _____ Hypernatremia (200 mEq/l)

(a) 12 ml/kg of 3% sodium chloride solution
(b) Peritoneal dialysis
(c) 3 mEq/kg/hour potassium, intravenously
(d) 0.2 mEq/kg solution of magnesium sulfate, intramuscularly
(e) Ion exchange resin, orally
(f) Rapid infusion of calcium gluconate

QUESTIONS 39–48

For each of the following statements, mark "A" if the statement is true about freshwater drowning, "B" if it is true about seawater drowning, "C" if it is true of both, "D" if it is true of neither.

39. _____ Lungs fill with fluid
40. _____ Hypoxemia most prominent sign
41. _____ Hyponatremia common
42. _____ Hyperchloremia common
43. _____ Metabolic acidosis
44. _____ Transient increase in blood volume
45. _____ Hemolysis
46. _____ Hypertonic fluid is the treatment of choice
47. _____ Corticosteroids will diminish damage
48. _____ Roentgenogram of the chest not immediately helpful

QUESTIONS 49–53

A 4-year-old boy (weight 15 kg, surface area 0.68 M^2) is brought to the emergency room with second- and third-degree burns of the trunk and back. The ambulance crew had started normal saline, 20 ml/kg/hour, intravenously, in the arm.

49. Initial physiologic reactions expected following severe burns include which *two* of the following?

(a) Diminished cardiac output
(b) Impaired myocardial contractility
(c) Decreased glomerular filtration rate
(d) Decreased secretion of antidiuretic hormone

50. On arrival at the emergency room, each of the following should be an *immediate* concern EXCEPT

(a) maintenance of airway
(b) evaluation of cardiac status

(c) maintenance of intravenous line
(d) inspection of wounds and search for unrecognized injuries
(e) calculation of extent of burns and fluid requirement for first 24 hours

51. Other important measures include each of the following EXCEPT

(a) insertion of Foley catheter
(b) insertion of nasogastric tube
(c) phenobarbital for sedation
(d) penicillin, intramuscularly
(e) tetanus toxoid, intramuscularly

52. In planning for fluids, electrolytes, and colloids for this patient, which one of the following is true?

(a) The appropriate amount of fluids is best calculated on a per-kg basis
(b) Total fluid in the first 24 hours should be 2000 ml/M² maintenance plus 5000 ml/M² additionally
(c) A total of 2720 ml of fluids should be administered in the first 12 hours
(d) 1360 ml of fluid should be given in the first 8 hours and 1360 ml in the next 16 hours
(e) Fluid management is best monitored by replacing urine output and insensible losses

53. The leading cause of death in burn patients after the initial 48 hours is

(a) renal failure
(b) sepsis
(c) cardiac failure
(d) pulmonary edema

QUESTIONS 54–57

A 12-month-old infant is admitted to the hospital because of dehydration and diarrhea of 3 days' duration. The infant weighed 10 kg at a well visit 1 week ago. She has had 10 to 12 stools per day for the last few days and a temperature of 39°C. She has not urinated for the past 18 hours. Physical examination reveals sunken eyes and dry, "tenting" skin.

54. Which of the following would you do first?

(a) Order a complete blood count and blood cultures

(b) Obtain a urine specimen for culture, electrolytes, and specific gravity
(c) Begin Ringer lactate, 20 ml/kg, intravenously, after obtaining blood for electrolytes and blood urea nitrogen
(d) Obtain stool for fats, reducing substances, and culture

55. If the child had been receiving only Kool-Aid for two days as "clear fluid" therapy, which electrolyte picture would you expect?

	Sodium mEq/l	Potassium mEq/l	Chloride mEq/l	Bicarbonate mEq/l
(a)	142	4.5	100	26
(b)	154	3.4	112	10
(c)	124	3.6	94	10
(d)	102	6.9	92	10

56. Had the mother given the child only boiled skimmed milk for the preceding 48 hours, which serum sodium level would you expect prior to therapy?

(a) 142 mEq/l
(b) 154 mEq/l
(c) 124 mEq/l
(d) 102 mEq/l

57. Assuming 10% dehydration, the best way to monitor initial improvement in this child is

(a) weight
(b) urinary output
(c) central venous pressure
(d) blood pressure

58. The most common cause of shock in the pediatric age group is

(a) hypovolemia secondary to hemorrhage or dehydration
(b) sepsis
(c) anaphylaxis
(d) CNS injury
(e) cardiac failure

59. Which of the following statements is true?

(a) Lifelong immunosuppression is required for recipients of autologous bone marrow transplantation
(b) Graft-versus-host disease does not occur in HLA-identical marrow transplants from siblings

(c) Survival of younger (< 2 years old) recipients of kidneys is better than that of adolescents

(d) Rejection of a transplanted liver usually occurs within the first few weeks and is unusual after 3 months

60. Which statement is true?

(a) Neonates do not feel pain

(b) Facial expression is the most reliable indicator of pain in infancy

(c) Opiates should not be used because of their addictive properties

(d) Exclusion of parents reduces the need for pharmacologic agents in pain management associated with procedures

61. In a descriptive definition of clinical pharmacology, which of the following is a pharmacodynamic parameter?

(a) Interaction with biologic receptors

(b) Absorption

(c) Distribution

(d) Excretion

62. When a patient is receiving phenytoin for a seizure disorder, the best indicator of therapeutic success is

(a) being seizure-free without toxic effects

(b) a maintenance dosage of 7 mg/kg daily

(c) serum drug levels in the therapeutic range

(d) serum drug levels in the therapeutic range and clinical seizure-free state

63. Adverse effects on the nursing infant may occur if the mother takes any of the following EXCEPT

(a) neomycin

(b) oral contraceptives

(c) reserpine

(d) atropine

(e) oral anticoagulants

64. Ultrasonography is commonly used to evaluate each of the following EXCEPT

(a) intracranial hemorrhage in neonates

(b) renal masses

(c) liver and biliary tract

(d) retroperitoneal and pelvic masses

(e) bone lesions

65. The radiation dose received by a child having a CT scan with contiguous slices approximates

(a) 0.001 Rad

(b) 0.01 Rad

(c) 0.1 Rad

(d) 1.0 Rad

(e) 10 Rads

66. Which of the following is likely to be the most useful diagnostic procedure in the clinical situation listed?

(a) CT scan in a child with headache

(a) MRI of skull in a 3-month-old with macrocephaly

(c) Barium swallow in a child with a suspected peptic ulcer

(d) IV Cholangiography in a child with suspected gallstones

7
Prenatal Disturbances

If you thought you left basic science behind with the last chapter's emphasis on physiology, welcome to the land of genetics. Actually, if you think you will ever be leaving basic science behind, perhaps you should go back to undergraduate school. If that depresses you, take heart. Pediatrics happens to be the best place to learn basic science, since children tend to have single pathologic conditions (if they have any at all, and most do not), and disease states tend to occur in their pure form.

Such is the case in the disturbances discussed in this chapter. Prenatal factors affecting childhood growth and development include genetics and environment. There has been an explosion of new knowledge in molecular genetics. The bulk of this chapter deals with the new and old genetics, with a practical guide toward genetic counseling included. So, with dim visions of Gregor Mendel and his peas, and the great Drosophila in the sky dancing in your head, see how you do with the following questions.

1. Each of the following is true of the human genome EXCEPT

(a) There are two copies in each somatic cell
(b) Most of the DNA in the genome appears to be represented by genes
(c) Most DNA is found in the nucleus of the cell
(d) Mitochondrial genes exhibit a maternal inheritance pattern
(e) There are many DNA sequences that appear to have no function.

2. Which of the following statements is true of mutations?

(a) They arise only in germ cells
(b) Missense mutations occur when a base is changed within the axon
(c) Polymorphisms result when mutations have significant impact on the health and functioning of an organism
(d) Translocations only occur in somatic cells

3. Each of the following genetic defects has been identified in man EXCEPT

(a) single mutant genes
(b) cytoplasmic inheritance
(c) chromosomal abnormalities
(d) multifactorial inheritance
(e) delayed mutation caused by environmental factors

4. Approximately what percentage of newborn infants have a hereditary malformation?

(a) 0.1–0.3%
(b) 0.5–0.8%
(c) 1–2%
(d) 3–5%

5. Which of the following statements most closely defines an allele?

(a) Two genes at homologous loci on their respective chromosomes
(b) A specific gene at a specific point on a single chromosome
(c) A gene having a specific effect on a heterozygous individual
(d) A gene having no effect on a heterozygous individual

QUESTIONS 6–17

For each of the following diseases, select the appropriate pattern of inheritance (a–d).

6. _____ Achondroplasia
7. _____ Sickle cell disease
8. _____ Phenylketonuria

(a) Autosomal recessive
(b) Autosomal dominant
(c) X-linked recessive

9. _____ Bruton hy-
pogamma-
globuline-
mia

10. _____ Color
blindness

11. _____ Polycystic
kidneys
(adult
type)

12. _____ Vitamin D-
resistant
rickets

13. _____ Tuberous
sclerosis

14. _____ Hurler syn-
drome

15. _____ Hemophilia
A (Factor
VIII defi-
ciency)

16. _____ Hemophilia
B (Factor
IX defi-
ciency)

17. _____ Duchenne
muscular
dystrophy

(d) X-linked domi-
nant

---

18. Which of the following statements regarding autosomal recessive inheritance is true?

    (a) The chances of two unrelated parents who are heterozygous for a condition passing that gene to an offspring is 25%.
    (b) The chance of disease being manifest in the offspring of two heterozygous parents is 50%.
    (c) Almost every human has several rare, harmful, recessive genes
    (d) Consanguinity quadruples the risk of birth defects

19. Each of the following statements regarding X-linked recessive diseases is true EXCEPT

    (a) Only males are affected
    (b) Affected sons may have an affected father
    (c) Only daughters are carriers
    (d) Affected sons may have an affected grandfather
    (e) Not all daughters of carrier mothers will be carriers

20. Which of the following statements about multifactorial inheritance is true?

    (a) Sex predilection does *not* occur
    (b) Identical twins are identically affected
    (c) There is a similar rate of recurrence among all first-degree relatives
    (d) The risk of abnormality is unrelated to the severity of the abnormality in relatives

21. The haploid number of chromosomes in the human is

    (a) 22
    (b) 23
    (c) 44
    (d) 46
    (e) 48

22. Human cells are said to be euploid if they

    (a) contain 23 chromosomes
    (b) contain 48 chromosomes
    (c) contain any exact multiple of the haploid number of chromosomes
    (d) are normal

23. The most common type of aneuploidy is

    (a) monosomy
    (b) diploidy
    (c) trisomy
    (d) polyploidy

24. Which of the following statements regarding aneupoidy is true?

    (a) Monosomy may result from metaphase lag
    (b) The incidence of nondisjunction is independent of maternal age
    (c) Pure polyploidy is rare, but some individuals with this condition have been identified
    (d) Nondisjunction occurring during mitotic division leads to mosaicism

25. Which of the following chromosomal structural aberrations is usually NOT associated with a phenotypic abnormality?

    (a) Deletion
    (b) Translocation
    (c) Reciprocal translocation
    (d) Ring chromosome
    (e) Centric fusion or robertsonian translocation

26. Which of the following is true about Down syndrome?

    (a) The increasing incidence of Down syndrome in children of younger women in recent years is a result of the increased incidence of infectious hepatitis

    (b) Translocation causes less than 5% of the cases of Down syndrome

    (c) Most cases of translocation Down syndrome are caused by inheritance from a carrier

    (d) Congenital heart disease is NOT a characteristic feature of Down syndrome

    (e) The risk of Down syndrome is as much as 1% in children of mothers 35 years of age

27. Superoxide dismutase is an enzyme whose gene locus is found on which chromosome?

    (a) 5
    (b) 13
    (c) 15
    (d) 18
    (e) 21

28. Increased maternal age is a factor in each of the following EXCEPT

    (a) 5p – deletion
    (b) 13-trisomy syndrome
    (c) 18-trisomy syndrome
    (d) 18p – deletion
    (e) 21-trisomy (Down syndrome)

29. Bloom syndrome, Fanconi pancytopenia syndrome, and ataxia telangiectasia are all

    (a) autosomal recessive diseases with a high frequency of chromosomal breaks and rearrangements

    (b) X-linked recessive diseases

    (c) associated with deletions

    (d) autosomal dominant diseases with an increased risk of leukemia

30. The Lyon hypothesis states that

    (a) each cell has one genetically active X chromosome

    (b) Barr bodies will not be seen in Turner syndrome (XO)

    (c) the active X chromosome is maternal in origin

    (d) females will be mosaic for heterozygous alleles located on the X chromosome

31. Each of the following statements about Turner syndrome is true EXCEPT

    (a) It is most frequently caused by monosomy of the X chromosome (i.e., karyotype 45, X)

    (b) It is associated with advanced maternal age

    (c) Risk of recurrence is NOT increased with the second child even if the first child is affected

    (d) Characteristic features include "streak" gonads and short stature

    (e) Mosaicism is a common characteristic

QUESTIONS 32–33

You are called to the delivery room to attend the delivery of an infant to a 39-year-old primigravida. The infant (infant A) is normal, but you notice syndactyly of the second and third toes bilaterally. Before you can talk with the mother, you are called across the hall to attend another delivery, this one a small for gestational age (38-week, 230-gram) infant (infant B) who has microcephaly, heart defects, jaundice, and cataracts.

32. What would you order for infant A?

    (a) Routine nursery care

    (b) Routine nursery care and roentgenograms of both feet

    (c) Routine nursery care, roentgenograms of both feet, and an orthopedic consultation

    (d) All of the above, plus genetic counseling for the parents

33. What would you order for infant B?

    (a) Routine nursery care

    (b) Isolation precautions and evaluation for congenital infection

    (c) Routine care and chromosomal studies and genetic counseling for the parents

    (d) Routine care and evaluation of mother for diabetes mellitus

---

34. Microcephaly is a feature of each of the following EXCEPT

    (a) congenital rubella
    (b) congenital cytomegalovirus infection
    (c) maternal alcoholism

(d) maternal thalidomide ingestion
(e) phenylketonuria

35. Teratogenic effects of each of the following occur primarily in the first trimester EXCEPT

   (a) thalidomide
   (b) rubella virus
   (c) estrogen
   (d) toxoplasma
   (e) tetracycline

36. Which of the following roentgenographic studies has the greatest potential danger to the pregnant woman?

   (a) Anteroposterior chest film
   (b) Flat plate of the abdomen
   (c) Intravenous pyelogram
   (d) Barium enema
   (e) Cholangiogram

37. Each of the following represents a single primary structural defect of prenatal onset EXCEPT

   (a) ventricular septal defect
   (b) cleft lip with cleft palate
   (c) Down syndrome
   (d) congenital hip dislocation
   (e) pyloric stenosis

QUESTIONS 38–40

For each of the following conditions, choose the appropriate matching karyotype (a-d).

38. _____ Macro-or-   (a) 45,X
          chidism   (b) 47,XXY
39. _____ Micro-or-   (c) 47,XXX
          chidism   (d) "Fragile-X" syn-
40. _____ Normal   drome
          fertility
          with no
          characteris-
          tic pheno-
          type

8

Inborn Errors of Metabolism

Whereas the last chapter reviewed basic genetics, this chapter is a biochemist's dream. It could be a nitpicker's dream too, with the complexity of the intermediary metabolism scheme offering myriad opportunities for impossible multiple choice questions. Well, good news! The following questions won't take as much advantage of you as they could. Somehow, neither of us should need to worry about the difference between 5-N-methyltetrahydrofolate methyl transferase deficiency and 5-10-N-methylene-tetrahydrofolate reductase deficiency. If we encounter it, we can look it up.

1. Pernicious vomiting is a characteristic of each of the following diseases EXCEPT

    (a) isovaleric acidemia
    (b) glycogen storage disease
    (c) phenylketonuria
    (d) methylmalonic acidemia
    (e) valinemia

2. Hepatomegaly and liver disease are presenting factors of each of the following EXCEPT

    (a) glycogen storage disease
    (b) Wilson disease
    (c) propionic acidemia
    (d) tryosinemia
    (e) galactosemia

3. Which one of the following statements about classic phenylketonuria (PKU) is true?

    (a) It occurs in 1 of 30,000 live births in the United States
    (b) Inheritance is autosomal dominant
    (c) Infants with PKU are clinically normal at birth
    (d) The diagnosis can be made by testing the newborn's urine with 10% ferric chloride
    (e) Dietary control need only be adhered to until age 2

4. The diagnosis of PKU can be confirmed by each of the following EXCEPT

    (a) elevated plasma phenylalanine level
    (b) normal plasma tyrosine

    (c) increased phenylpyruvic acid in the urine
    (d) inability to tolerate orally administered phenylalanine
    (e) phenotype of blond hair and blue eyes

5. Which one of the following statements concerning tyrosinemia type I is true?

    (a) A transient form exists, primarily in premature infants, which responds to vitamin C therapy
    (b) Urine turns black on standing
    (c) Albinism occurs in most forms of the disease
    (d) Liver damage occurs in all forms of the disease
    (e) The disease is autosomal dominant with variable penetrance

QUESTIONS 6–11

For each disease, select the substance for which there is an error in metabolism (a–e).

6. ____ Hartnup disease	(a) Histidine
7. ____ Alcaptonuria	(b) Valine
8. ____ Oculocutaneous albinism	(c) Tryptophan
	(d) Tyrosine
9. ____ Indicanuria	(e) Cystine
10. ____ Maple syrup urine disease	
11. ____ Richner-Hanhart syndrome	

12. Each of the following is true of classic homocystinuria EXCEPT

(a) It is due to an inborn error of methionine metabolism—a deficiency of cystathionine synthetase
(b) It is autosomal recessive
(c) It occurs approximately in 1 of every 200,000 live births
(d) Ectopia lentis is presenting symptom
(e) Folic acid in high doses causes clinical improvement

13. On routine urinalysis an otherwise normal 6-year-old child is found to have many oxalate crystals. The most likely diagnosis is

(a) pyridoxine deficiency
(b) ethylene glycol ingestion
(c) primary hyperoxaluria
(d) spinach or rhubarb intake

14. Each of the following enzymes participates in the Krebs-Henseleit (urea) cycle EXCEPT

(a) ornithine transcarbamylase
(b) carbamyl phosphate synthetase
(c) argininosuccinic acid synthetase
(d) argininosuccinase
(e) histidase

QUESTIONS 15–20

For each inborn error of amino acid metabolism, select the correct urine odor (a–g).

15. _____ Glutaric acidemia (type II)
16. _____ Phenylketonuria
17. _____ Methionine malabsorption
18. _____ Trimethylaminuria
19. _____ Oasthouse disease
20. _____ Hawkinsuria

(a) Cabbage
(b) Hoplike
(c) Sweaty feet
(d) Rotting fish
(e) Mousy
(f) Swimming pool
(g) Maple syrup

21. Which of the following is the most common disorder of intramitochondrial oxidation?

(a) Electron-transfer flavoprotein deficiency
(b) Medium-chain acyl-CoA dehydrogenase deficiency
(c) Glutaric aciduria, type II
(d) Carnitine palmityl transferase deficiency

22. Zellweger syndrome is a disorder of

(a) long-chain acyl-CoA dehydrogenase
(b) peroxisome biogenesis
(c) lipoprotein transport
(d) lysosomal storage

23. Tay Sachs disease is an example of a

(a) G_{M1} gangliosidosis
(b) G_{M2} gangliosidosis
(c) mucopolysaccharidosis
(d) mucolipidosis

24. The enzymatic defect in Fabry disease is

(a) α-galactosidase
(b) α-fucosidase
(c) α-hexosaminidase
(d) β-hexosaminidase

25. Each of the following is a finding in Gaucher disease EXCEPT

(a) massive splenomegaly
(b) hepatomegaly
(c) only observed in Ashkenazi Jews
(d) central nervous system degeneration
(e) PAS- and acid phosphatase-positive cells in bone marrow

26. Each of the following disorders is characterized by neurologic degeneration EXCEPT

(a) Farber disease
(b) Niemann-Pick disease
(c) metachromatic leukodystrophy
(d) Krabbe disease

27. Which of the following is true about serum cholesterol normal values?

(a) The decrease in the neonatal period represents a loss of LDL
(b) The levels in boys are significantly higher than in girls
(c) The increase in adulthood is due almost entirely to an increase in LDL
(d) HDL levels drop in females during the second decrease

28. Each of the following is true of a "prudent diet" EXCEPT

(a) 30% of total calories as fat
(b) No more than 100 mg cholesterol/1000 calories

(c) Maximum 300 mg cholesterol intake/24 hours

(d) Useful for any child with hyperlipidemia

29. An infant with diarrhea tolerates milk well, but gets worse with fruit juices and Kool-Aid. The most likely enzyme deficiency is

(a) lactase
(b) maltase
(c) sucrose-isomaltase
(d) amylase

30. Which statement is true about late-onset lactose intolerance?

(a) There is a high incidence in black Americans
(b) Cases are generally severe
(c) Approximately 10% of northern European people are affected
(d) Fruit juices and many other clear fluids exacerbate symptoms

QUESTIONS 31–33

An infant has chronic diarrhea and failure to thrive. The stool is tested with Clinitest tablets and glucose oxidase strips. For each of the lab results below, select the most likely enzyme deficiency (a–d).

(a) Maltase
(b) Lactase
(c) Sucrase (stool unhydrolyzed)
(d) Sucrase (stool hydrolyzed)

	Cupric sulfate (Clinitest)	Glucose oxidase
31. _____	+	−
32. _____	−	−
33. _____	+	+

34. Which enzyme deficiency is responsible for classic galactosemia?

(a) Galactokinase
(b) Galactose-1-phosphate uridyl transferase
(c) Uridyl diphosphate galactose 4-epimerase
(d) Glucose-6-phosphatase

35. The build-up of galactose-1-phosphate causes each of the following symptoms of galactosemia EXCEPT

(a) cataracts
(b) hepatic cirrhosis
(c) mental retardation
(d) ascites and splenomegaly

36. Lactic acidosis that is clinically significant is associated with which type of glycogen storage disease?

(a) Type I
(b) Type IIa
(c) Type IV
(d) Type V
(e) Type IX

37. Which of the following forms of glycogen storage disease is sex-linked recessive instead of autosomal recessive?

(a) I
(b) IIa
(c) VII
(d) IXb
(e) X

38. Precise diagnosis of infants with defects in carbohydrate metabolism relies most on which of the following?

(a) Serum lactate and pyruvate levels
(b) Urinary excretion of catecholamines
(c) Ultrasound measurement of heart and liver
(d) Tissue analysis

QUESTIONS 39–45

For each of the following, mark "A" if heparan sulfate is found in the urine, "B" if dermatan sulfaturia is present, "C" if both are present, "D" if neither is present.

39. _____ Hurler syndrome
40. _____ Hunter syndrome
41. _____ Scheie syndrome
42. _____ Morquio syndrome A
43. _____ Sanfilippo syndrome A
44. _____ Morquio syndrome B
45. _____ Maroteaux-Lamy syndrome

46. Each of the following statements about gout is true EXCEPT

(a) It is primarily a disease of males
(b) A complete deficiency of hypoxanthine guanine phosphoribosyltransferase leads to Lesch-Nyhan syndrome
(c) High uric acid levels fall with steady work
(d) It is found in patients with type II glycogen storage disease

47. Self-destructive behavior is a component of

(a) xanthinuria
(b) Lesch-Nyhan syndrome
(c) orotic aciduria
(d) adenosine deaminase deficiency

48. The Hoesch test, when positive, is diagnostic for

(a) hemochromatosis
(b) methemoglobinemia
(c) acute intermittent prophyria
(d) Gaucher disease

QUESTIONS 49–55

For each question, choose as many answers as appropriate. *One or more than one* may be correct.

49. Which of the following statements about Type I (insulin-dependent or juvenile-onset) diabetes mellitus is/are true?

(a) American blacks have a higher incidence than Caucasians
(b) It is most likely to begin at ages 5 to 7 and at puberty
(c) The incidence is significantly higher in boys than in girls
(d) Most cases have their onset in the summer months
(e) Approximately 1% of children will develop juvenile-onset diabetes

50. Which of the following statements regarding the etiology of Type I diabetes mellitus (IDDM) is/are true?

(a) A high glucose intake can lead to IDDM
(b) The disease is inherited in an autosomal recessive manner
(c) Viral infections and autoimmune inflammatory reactions are implicated in genetically predisposed individuals

(d) Extreme exertion causing hypoglycemia can result in IDDM
(e) The pathogenesis of IDDM is similar to that of maturity-onset diabetes mellitus

51. Which of the following is/are likely in the blood of a child who has just been diagnosed as having diabetes mellitus?

(a) Absent insulin
(b) Elevated glucose
(c) Elevated triglycerides
(d) Low cholesterol
(e) Elevated glucagon

52. Which statements is/are true about the natural history of Type I diabetes mellitus?

(a) Most patients are first seen in diabetic coma
(b) A small number of children will have a partial remission from their insulin requirement within 2 to 3 months of the onset
(c) Insulin requirements are hardest to determine during the intensification phase
(d) In the permanent diabetic state, day-to-day variability in the insulin requirement is diminished
(e) Insulin requirements decrease after adolescence

53. The diagnosis of Type I (IDDM) diabetes mellitus cannot be made unless which of the following is/are present?

(a) Unexplained hyperglycemia
(b) Renal glycosuria
(c) Ketonemia
(d) Ketonuria
(e) Metabolic acidosis

54. Attainable objectives in the long-term management of diabetes mellitus include

(a) elimination of polyuria, polydipsia, and polyphagia
(b) normal growth and development
(c) continuously normal serum glucose levels
(d) an HbA_{rc} fraction of 6 to 9%
(e) prevention of microvascular disease

55. Which of the following insulin preparations has/have onset of action at 2 hours and peak effect at between 4 to 12 hours?

(a) NPH
(b) Lente

(c) Regular
(d) Ultralente
(e) Protamine zinc insulin (PZI)

---

56. Which statement is true about hypoglycemic reactions in diabetic children?

    (a) The onset is insidious
    (b) Symptoms include thirst, dry mouth, and trembling
    (c) They have been implicated in provoking epileptic seizures
    (d) "Diet" sodas should be readily available for aborting attacks
    (e) Exercise and insulin requirements should be increased to prevent recurrences

57. Which of the following findings should alert one to the possibility of the Somogyi phenomenon in a diabetic child? (Choose as many as are appropriate.)

    (a) Persistent ketonuria without ketoacidosis
    (b) Frequent nightmares
    (c) Persistent hyperglycemia
    (d) Excessive sweating at night
    (e) Diabetic dwarfism

58. Associated endocrinopathies commonly seen in children with diabetes include (choose as many as are appropriate)

    (a) parathyroid disorders
    (b) Addison disease
    (c) hypothyroidism
    (d) ovarian failure
    (e) myasthenia gravis

QUESTIONS 59–68

You receive an 11 PM call from a father who just came home and found his 16-year-old diabetic daughter semiconscious on the living room couch. He tells you that she seemed depressed for a week since she "broke up" with her steady boyfriend of 1 year.

59. Which of the following should you ask? (Choose as many as appropriate.)

    (a) Has she taken her insulin today?
    (b) Is she cold and perspiring heavily?
    (c) is there any evidence of drug overdose?
    (d) Has she been ill?
    (e) Is there any evidence of head trauma?

60. It turns out that she is not cold and clammy, but rather hot and dry. There is no evidence of drugs or trauma, and she has been well. He doesn't know whether or not she took her insulin. What should you tell him to do now? (Choose one.)

    (a) Give her some oral glucose, then bring her to the hospital
    (b) Give her an insulin injection at twice the usual daily dose, and call you again in two hours
    (c) Give her syrup of ipecac and bring her to the hospital
    (d) Bring her to the hospital immediately
    (e) Give her two aspirins and call you back in the morning

61. When you finally see her she is stuporous and breathing rapidly and deeply at a rate of 40 per minute. She appears very dehydrated, and her skin is dry and warm. Which of the following should be done immediately? (Choose as many as are appropriate.)

    (a) Begin intravenous administration of normal saline at 20 ml/kg over a 45-minute period
    (b) Administer insulin, 2.0 units/kg subcutaneously
    (c) Order serum glucose, electrolytes, and arterial blood pH determinations
    (d) Order a toxicology screen
    (e) Start intravenous administration of insulin at 0.1 units/kg by rapid push

The results of the laboratory work are as follows:

Serum glucose	640 mg/dl
Serum electrolytes:	
Sodium	134 mEq/l
Potassium	3.2 mEq/l
Chloride	105 mEq/l
Bicarbonate	7 mEq/l
Arterial blood pH	7.12

For each of the possible therapeutic measures for this patient (42–48), select the lettered answer (a–e) that represents the correct timing. (Assume that she weighs 50 kg.) Note: Each lettered answer may be appropriate for one, more than one, or none of the numbered items.

62. _____ Begin regular insulin, subcutaneously

    (a) Within the first 2 hours of treatment

63. _____ Replace calculated fluid deficit
64. _____ Replace potassium as phosphate
65. _____ Replace potassium as chloride
66. _____ Give at least 120 mEq of sodium bicarbonate
67. _____ Administer 5% glucose in 0.2% saline with 20 mEq/l potassium chloride as basic fluid
68. _____ Begin a clear fluid diet

(b) During the first 6 to 8 hours of treatment
(c) Between 8 and 24 hours after initiation of treatment
(d) One the second day of treatment
(e) At any time

---

69. Which of the following statements about hypoglycemia is/are true?

(a) Leucine-sensitive individuals develop hypoglycemia as a result of hyperinsulinism
(b) The transfusion of acid citrate dextrose (ACD) blood may lead to hypoglycemia
(c) Serum insulin levels are greatly elevated in Reye syndrome, causing a profound hypoglycemia
(d) Hepatic enzyme deficiencies leading to hypoglycemia are all autosomal recessive diseases
(e) Glucagon is effective in eliminating hypoglycemia in glycogen storage disease

70. Which of the following statements about ketotic hypoglycemia is/are true?

(a) Onset is usually between 6 and 12 months of age
(b) Attacks usually occur first thing in the morning or after a fast
(c) The disease spontaneously disappears in most patients by 10 years of age
(d) Most patients with ketotic hypoglycemia also have panhypopituitarism
(e) Between attacks, carbohydrate tolerance tests give normal results

9

The Fetus and the Neonatal Infant

No area of pediatrics has grown more rapidly during last 20 years than neonatology. In the 1940s and 1950s, nurseries were part of the obstetrical service in most hospitals. Pediatricians were asked occasionally to come discharge an infant or to calculate the proper formula if there was prematurity or some other complication. In the 1960s it was rare for a sick 1500-gram infant to survive. Now it is rare for such an infant to die, and 750-gram infants are successfully developing into normal children.

This chapter in the textbook comprehensively develops the science and technology of the care of the fetus and newborn. Many aspects of neonatology are also covered elsewhere in the text (e.g., rubella, cytomegalovirus, hypoglycemia), yet there are often special problems associated with these disorders as they affect the newborn full-term or premature infant. That is the focus of these questions, and most of them will test you on those aspects of disease that are unique to the neonate. A few patient management problems are interspersed, with a comprehensive one at the end. Have fun, and if you find this chapter frustrating, remember that it is easier than starting an IV on a 750-gram infant.

1. Each of the following is true regarding neonatal mortality rate (NMR) in the United States EXCEPT

   (a) The NMR is higher for black children than for white children
   (b) The NMR has progressively declined for all infants over the past decade
   (c) The NMR for white infants is approximately 4/1000 while it is 10/1000 for black infants
   (d) The NMR is higher in the United States than in Scandanavia, Japan, and the Netherlands
   (e) The NMR is highest in the first 24 hours of life and composes 65% of infant deaths under a year

2. What percentage of pregnant patients are "high risk" on the basis of their medical history?

   (a) 1 to 5%
   (b) 5 to 10%
   (c) 10 to 20%
   (d) 20 to 40%

3. The lowest neonatal mortality rate occurs in which maternal age group?

   (a) 15 to 20 years
   (b) 20 to 30 years
   (c) 30 to 35 years
   (d) 35 to 45 years

4. Ultrasound is useful for each of the following EXCEPT

   (a) estimation of fetal size
   (b) determining the placental location
   (c) estimation of fetal maturity and risk of hyaline membrane disease
   (d) recognition of anencephaly
   (e) diagnosing intrauterine growth retardation

5. Each of the following statements is true about the L/S ratio EXCEPT

   (a) It approaches 2:1 at about 25 weeks' gestation
   (b) Maternal diabetes will be associated with a lower ratio
   (c) Meconium contamination will reduce the reliability of the test
   (d) 90 to 95% of infants with a radio of less than 2:1 will develop hyaline membrane disease
   (e) Fetal blood contamination will not invalidate the result

6. Which one of the following statements is true?

    (a) Assuming healthy mothers at term, neonatal mortality rates are lowest (~0.3%) when labors last less than 24 hours

    (b) Delivery by cesarean section carries no greater risk to the infant than does vaginal delivery

    (c) Polyhydramnios is associated with renal hypoplasia

    (d) Midforceps deliveries are associated with an increased frequency of anoxic incidents in the newborn

7. Which one of the following physical findings is abnormal in the newborn?

    (a) Mongolian spots
    (b) Craniotabes
    (c) Wormian bones
    (d) Epstein pearls

8. An infant has the following findings at 5 minutes: pulse 130 per minute, cyanotic hands and feet, good muscle tone, and a strong cry and grimace. This infant's Apgar score is

    (a) 7
    (b) 8
    (c) 9
    (d) 10

9. Newborns (term or premature) should be given each of the following prophylactic measures EXCEPT

    (a) daily hexachlorophene baths
    (b) triple dye to cord
    (c) silver nitrate to eyes
    (d) vitamin K, intramuscularly

10. Which of the following drugs are *absolutely* contraindicated in nursing mothers? (More than one answer may be correct.)

    (a) Propranolol
    (b) Methadone
    (c) Chloramphenicol
    (d) Immunosuppressants
    (e) Propylthiouracil

11. Which infant has the lowest risk for neonatal mortality?

    (a) 2400-gram, 36-week gestation
    (b) 2400-gram, 40-week gestation
    (c) 3600-gram, 35-week gestation
    (d) 3000-gram, 38-week gestation
    (e) 4500-gram, 42-week gestation

12. Which of the following statements is true about twinning?

    (a) Twins of the same sex are always dizygotic
    (b) The incidence of twinning is higher in Oriental people than in blacks
    (c) Monozygotic twins may have dichorionic placentas
    (d) Perinatal mortality is only minimally (< twofold) higher

13. Which of the following is not generally considered as a cause of death in a 1500-gram infant?

    (a) Prematurity
    (b) Sepsis
    (c) Anoxia
    (d) Hyaline membrane disease
    (e) Intraventricular hemorrhage

14. Very low birthweight infants (choose the correct answer)

    (a) are as likely to be black as white
    (b) account for the overwhelming majority of neonatal deaths
    (c) are less than 1500 grams and predominantly premature
    (d) are usually small for gestational age

15. Which of the following infants are LEAST likely to develop hypoglycemia?

    (a) Premature infants who are small for gestational age
    (b) Premature infants whose size is appropriate for gestational age (1800 to 2000 grams)
    (c) Term infants who are small for gestational age
    (d) Infants of diabetic mothers who are premature and large for gestational age

16. Incubators are important in the care of premature infants for each of the following reasons EXCEPT

    (a) maintenance of neutral thermal environment
    (b) oxygen administration
    (c) maintenance of correct relative humidity
    (d) infection control in the nursery

17. Each of the following is an acceptable method for feeding premature infants EXCEPT

(a) gastrostomy tube
(b) nasogastric gavage
(c) bottle
(d) breast

18. Infants on total parenteral nutrition may develop azotemia and dehydration. This is usually a result of which one of the following?

(a) Hypoglycemia
(b) Hyperglycemia
(c) Hyperammonemia
(d) Hyperchloremic acidosis
(e) Miscalculation of fluid requirements

19. Which of the following is the most important factor in the successful care of a premature infant?

(a) The skill, availability, and experience of the nursing staff
(b) The training and experience of the pediatrician
(c) The availability of monitors, respirators, and other equipment
(d) The avoidance of infection

20. Neonatal cyanosis is seen in each of the following EXCEPT

(a) meningitis
(b) hypoglycemia
(c) respiratory disease
(d) cardiac right-to-left shunt
(e) hemorrhagic shock

21. Fever in neonates is most often a sign of which of the following?

(a) Overdressing or overheating
(b) Viral infection
(c) Bacterial infection
(d) Dehydration

22. Sepsis in neonates is often accompanied by each of the following EXCEPT

(a) fever
(b) failure to feed well
(c) irritability
(d) jaundice
(e) lethargy

23. A 1-week-old infant is brought to the emergency room because of vomiting and diarrhea for 2 days. His mother tells you that he is taking formula vigorously and urinating well ("wet all the time"). He looks alert. The most likely diagnosis is

(a) sepsis
(b) gastroenteritis
(c) malrotation of the intestine
(d) midgut volvulus
(e) overfeeding

24. A newborn is noted to have a right parietal cephalohematoma. Which suture lines does the swelling obliterate?

(a) Sagittal
(b) Parietal
(c) Occipital
(d) Coronal
(e) None of the above

QUESTIONS 25–27

For each paralytic syndrome, select the involved nerve(s) (a–d).

25. _____ Klumpke paralysis   (a) Fifth and sixth cervical
26. _____ Erb-Duchenne paralysis   (b) Seventh and eighth cervical, first thoracic
27. _____ Facial nerve palsy   (c) Phrenic
   (d) Seventh cranial

28. Which bone is most often fractured in difficult deliveries?

(a) Clavicle
(b) Humerus
(c) Radius
(d) Femur
(e) Tibia

29. An infant in the delivery room is noted to have respiratory movements but no air is entering the lungs with the mouth closed. The most likely diagnosis is

(a) narcosis
(b) choanal atresia
(c) diaphragmatic hernia
(d) pulmonary hypoplasia
(e) congenital heart disease

30. Which of the following statements about apnea in the neonatal period is true?

    (a) Apnea is always a sign of sepsis in premature infants
    (b) Apnea does *not* occur in normal term infants.
    (c) Physical stimulation is useful in the management of term infants only
    (d) Apnea in a premature infant is a predictor of sudden infant death syndrome
    (e) Increased humidity and theophylline have been found to reduce the number of apneic episodes in premature infants

31. Which of the following statements about hyaline membrane disease is NOT true?

    (a) The incidence is inversely proportional to gestational age and birth weight
    (b) There is an increased frequency in infants of diabetic mothers
    (c) Surfactant in the pulmonary alveolar lining is deficient
    (d) A lack of surfactant leads to atelectasis and severe ventilation-perfusion abnormalities
    (e) Death occurs within 3 days in all but mild cases

32. Which of the following is an indication for the use of continuous positive airway pressure in the treatment of an infant with hyaline membrane disease?

    (a) Hypercarbia and hypoxia on room air
    (b) Hypoxemia on 70% oxygen
    (c) Hypoxemia and hypercarbia on 100% oxygen
    (d) Cyanosis and hypotension

33. Which of the following is an indication for the use of assisted ventilation in an infant with hyaline membrane disease?

    (a) Cyanoisis and hypotension
    (b) Hypoxemia, hypercarbia, and metabolic acidosis on 70% oxygen
    (c) Hypoxemia, hypercarbia, and metabolic acidosis on 100% oxygen
    (d) Apneic episodes without bradycardia

34. Complications of treatment for hyaline membrane disease include each of the following EXCEPT

    (a) retrolental fibroplasia
    (b) bronchopulmonary dysplasia

    (c) vascular embolization
    (d) pulmonary artery stenosis
    (e) subglottic stenosis

35. Which of the following statements is true regarding extracorporeal membrane oxygenation (ECMO)?

    (a) It is available routinely for infants with severe hyaline membrane disease
    (b) Infants under 2.0 kg can be safely treated
    (c) 85 to 90% of infants with persistent fetal circulation survive
    (d) Ventilator therapy must be continued at approximately the same rate, pressure, and oxygenation

36. A newborn infant is tachypneic and has prominent pulmonary vascular markings, flat diaphragms, and fluid in the fissures. There is no hypoxemia, hypercarbia, or acidosis. Which of the following is most likely?

    (a) Hyaline membrane disease
    (b) Meconium aspiration
    (c) Pneumomediastinum
    (d) Transient tachypnea of the newborn
    (e) Wilson-Mekity syndrome

37. Bile-stained vomitus in a newborn is most likely to be the result of which of the following?

    (a) Esophageal atresia
    (b) Pyloric stenosis
    (c) Chalasia
    (d) Midgut volvulus

38. Meconium plug may be an early sign of which of the following?

    (a) Pyloric stenosis
    (b) Congenital aganglionic megacolon
    (c) Malrotation
    (d) Intestinal perforation

39. Each statement about necrotizing enterocolitis (NEC) is true EXCEPT

    (a) Incidence is 1 to 5% of admissions to neonatal intensive care units
    (b) Rotovirus is the etiologic agent
    (c) Perinatal stress is a predisposing factor
    (d) Diagnosis depends on a high level of suspicion
    (e) Medical management is successful in 80% of cases

40. Jaundice is most likely to be "physiologic" in a term infant in which one of the following situations?

(a) Jaundice at 12 hours of age
(b) Serum bilirubin increasing 5 mg/dl/24 hours or less in the first 2 to 4 days
(c) Direct (conjugated) serum bilirubin greater than 1 mg/dl
(d) Jaundice at 12 days of age

41. Which of the following is most appropriate for treating hyperbilirubinemia (11.2 mg/dl) in a 3-week-old and breast-fed infant with normal growth and development?

(a) Phototherapy
(b) Exchange transfusion
(c) Phenobarbital
(d) None of the above

42. Opisthotonos, bulging fontanelle, lethargy, poor feeding, and a high-pitched cry are found in each of the following EXCEPT

(a) intracranial hemorrhage
(b) sepsis
(c) kernicterus
(d) asphyxia
(e) hypothyroidism

43. Which of the following is a necessary prerequisite for the "bronze baby" syndrome?

(a) Kernicterus
(b) Phototherapy
(c) High indirect (unconjugated) serum bilirubin
(d) Hepatitis
(e) Carotenemia

44. Which of the following infants should receive immediate exchange transfusions?

(a) A normal, full-term, 4-day-old infant whose serum bilirubin is 20 mg/dl
(b) A preterm, 8-day-old baby with no complications whose serum bilirubin is 19 mg/dl
(c) A 2-day-old term infant with Rh incompatibility whose serum bilirubin is 16 mg/dl
(d) A 4-week-old breast-fed infant whose serum bilirubin is 12 mg/dl

45. Each of the following is a cause of anemia in the first few days of life EXCEPT

(a) hemolytic disease of the newborn (erythroblastosis fetalis)

(b) congenital spherocytosis
(c) cephalhematoma
(d) intrauterine hemorrhage

46. Which of the following antigens is most often associated with significant hemolytic disease?

(a) C (Rh)
(b) D (Rh)
(c) E (Rh)
(d) K (Kell)
(e) Duffy

47. Which of the following statements about Rh incompatibility is true?

(a) Spontaneous abortion frequently results in sensitization of mothers
(b) Rh disease in infants is *not* related to birth order
(c) If a mother and infant are incompatible for both ABO and Rh factors, the disease is doubly severe
(d) Exchange transfusion is the best method for preventing the disease

48. Which of the following is LEAST likely in a 1-hour-old infant with moderate Rh incompatibility?

(a) Anemia
(b) Positive direct Coombs test
(c) Jaundice
(d) Reticulocytosis

49. Which of the following should be used for IMMEDIATE exchange transfusion in a severely hydropic infant?

(a) Type O, Rh negative whole blood
(b) Type O, Rh positive whole blood
(c) Type-specific (A, B, or AB) Rh-negative whole blood
(d) Type-specific Rh-positive whole blood

50. Which of the following is true of ABO incompatibility?

(a) It is caused by IgM isoantibodies
(b) It is less severe than Rh incompatibility
(c) It does *not* occur in first-born children
(d) It is less common than Rh incompability

51. Which of the following blood factors are decreased in the newborn?

(a) II, VII, IX, and X
(b) II, V, VII, and IX

(c) V, VII, IX, and X
(d) VII, VIII, IX, and XI

52. Hemorrhagic disease of the newborn is effectively prevented by which of the following?

(a) Infusion of fresh frozen plasma
(b) Injection of anti-D globulin (RhoGAM) in the mother
(c) Injection of 1 mg vitamin K at birth
(d) Heparin
(e) Platelet transfusion

53. The Apt test takes advantage of which biochemical fact?

(a) Adult hemoglobin in alkali resistant
(b) Fetal hemoglobin in alkali resistant
(c) Sickle hemoglobin in alkali resistant
(d) Rh-sensitized cells are alkali resistant

54. A clear, light-yellow discharge from the umbilicus of a newborn is indicative of which one of the following?

(a) Patency of the omphalomesenteric duct
(b) A urachal cyst
(c) A congenital omphalocele
(d) An umbilical granuloma

55. Most umbilical hernias

(a) resolve spontaneously
(b) need strapping
(c) require elective surgery
(d) require immediate surgery

56. Each of the following statements is true about neonatal hypomagnesemia EXCEPT

(a) It is usually associated with hypocalcemia
(b) Clinical signs occur when the serum level drops below 1.2 mg/dl
(c) Tetany unresponsive to calcium should be treated with magnesium
(d) It is treated with intramuscular magnesium sulfate
(e) It commonly occurs following the treatment of eclampsia in the mother

QUESTIONS 57–58

A 2100-gram, full-term infant becomes irritable and develops coarse tremors at 36 hours of age. He feeds poorly and has diarrhea and nasal stuffiness.

57. Which one of the following is the most likely diagnosis?

(a) Hypocalcemia
(b) Hypomagnesemia
(c) Pyridoxine deficiency
(d) Heroin withdrawal from an addicted mother
(e) Hypoglycemia

58. The most appropriate treatment for this infant is

(a) 10% of calcium gluconate by slow intravenous infusion
(b) magnesium sulfate, intramuscularly
(c) pyridoxine pyrophosphate, intramuscularly
(d) phenobarbital, orally or intramuscularly
(e) 10% glucose in water, intravenously

---

59. Each of the following statements concerning infants of diabetic mothers is true EXCEPT

(a) Most of them are large for gestational age
(b) Hypoglycemia often occurs shortly after birth
(c) Tachypnea is common
(d) The incidence of hyaline membrane disease is the same as in matched controls of comparable gestational age

60. Each of the following is a predisposing factor to hypoglycemia in newborns EXCEPT

(a) diabetes in the mother
(b) very low birth weight
(c) small size for gestational age
(d) galactosemia
(e) hypoparathyroidism

61. Which of the following statements about infection in the neonatal period is true?

(a) Premature rupture of membranes less than 24 hours before delivery usually results in amnionitis
(b) Prematurity is the most important predisposing factor for neonatal infection
(c) Mother-to-fetus transmission of viral disease can occur even if the mother is immune
(d) Neonatal sepsis and urinary tract infection occur with equal frequency

62. Each of the following organisms infects the fetus by the transplacental route EXCEPT

    (a) rubella virus
    (b) chlamydia
    (c) *Toxoplasma gondii*
    (d) *Treponema pallidum*
    (e) cytomegalovirus

63. Which of the following infections in a neonate is usually associated with symptomatic disease in the mother?

    (a) Hepatitis B
    (b) Herpes genitalis (HSV-2)
    (c) Cytomegalovirus
    (d) Rubella virus

64. In order to diagnose congenital infection in a newborn by serologic means, which of the following sera are necessary?

    (a) Newborn and 3-month samples on infant; 3-month sample on mother for IgM
    (b) Newborn sample on infant and mother for IgG
    (c) Newborn and 3-month sample on infant; sample on mother at birth for IgG
    (d) Newborn and 3-month sample on infant; paired samples from the mother at the same time for IgG

65. Each of the following is necessary in dealing with a nursery epidemic of *Staphylococcus aureus* EXCEPT

    (a) cultures of all infants and personnel
    (b) isolation of colonized infants from uncolonized admissions
    (c) appropriate parenteral or topical antibiotics
    (d) cultures of water faucets, drains, and sink traps

66. The two most common etiologic agents for neonatal sepsis or meningitis are

    (a) *Staphylococcus aureus* and *Escherichia coli*
    (b) *Streptococcus pneumoniae* and *Haemophilus influenzae*
    (c) *Escherichia coli* and group B streptococcus
    (d) *Escherichia coli* and group A streptococcus
    (e) *Pseudomonas* and *Klebsiella* species

67. In the diagnostic evaluation of sepsis, MINIMUM cultures should include which of the following?

    (a) 0.5 to 1.0 ml blood and urine
    (b) Blood cultures ($\times 2$), cerebrospinal fluid, and urine
    (c) Throat, ear, nasopharynx, stool, and urine
    (d) 0.5 to 1.0 ml blood, urine, and cerebrospinal fluid

68. The most appropriate initial antibiotic regimen for treatment of neonatal sepsis while awaiting culture and sensitivity results is

    (a) penicillin and sulfacetamide
    (b) ampicillin and gentamicin
    (c) erythromycin and kanamycin
    (d) nafcillin and gentamicin
    (e) erythromycin and gentamicin

69. The prevention of sepsis (group B streptococci) in the neonate relies currently on which of the following?

    (a) The use of prophylactic antibiotics in mothers
    (b) The use of prophylactic antibiotics in newborns
    (c) Development of vaccines effective against group B streptococci for use in mothers
    (d) Development of vaccines effective against group B streptococci for use in newborns

70. The most common cause of osteomyelitis in a neonate is

    (a) *Streptococcus pyogenes* (group A)
    (b) *Escherichia coli*
    (c) *Staphylococcus aureus*
    (d) Anaerobic organisms

71. Urinary tract infection in newborns

    (a) is more common in males than females (3:1)
    (b) is most often associated with polycystic kidney disease
    (c) is usually caused by *Escherichia coli*
    (d) causes frequency and crying on urination

72. The most important historical fact in assessing whether neonatal conjunctivitis is chemical or infectious is

(a) timing of onset of conjunctivitis
(b) maternal history of gonococcal infection
(c) use of antibiotics in mother
(d) unresponsiveness to ophthalmologic topical antibiotics

73. Each of the following is true about otitis media in the neonate EXCEPT

(a) Preterm infants are affected more often than full-term infants
(b) *Streptococcus pneumoniae* and *Haemophilus influenzae* are the usual pathogens
(c) Symptoms are nonspecific
(d) Therapy is as for sepsis

QUESTIONS 74–79

For each of the following, mark "A" if the finding is associated with early-onset group B streptococcal disease, "B" if it is associated with late-onset disease, "C" if both, or "D" if neither.

74. _____ Respiratory distress in first 12 hours
75. _____ Organism responsive to penicillin
76. _____ Prevention with penicillin feasible
77. _____ Extremely high mortality
78. _____ Meningitis a feture
79. _____ Premature rupture of membranes.

80. Each is a common mode of cytomegalovirus transmission EXCEPT

(a) blood transfusion
(b) breast milk
(c) transplacentally
(d) nosocomially

81. Infants born to mothers with hepatitis B should

(a) not be at risk if they are breast-fed
(b) receive hepatitis B immune globulin
(c) not be discharged until free of hepatitis B antigen
(d) be carefully examined for congenital malformations

82. Which one of the following statements about neonatal herpes simplex is true?

(a) Disease is usually associated with oral or genital herpes, even if the mother is asymptomatic
(b) The onset is usually within 12 to 24 hours of birth
(c) Involvement of the central nervous system in the absence of skin lesions is common
(d) Cytosine arabinoside (ara-C) and iododeoxyuridine have been used successfully to treat the disease in neonates

83. Enteroviral disease in neonates is most often

(a) caused by polio viruses
(b) congenital in origin
(c) seen during the summer
(d) accompanied by meningitis

84. Varicella-zoster infection is most severe

(a) in utero
(b) at 0 to 4 days of age
(c) at 5 to 10 days of age
(d) in infants 3 to 6 months of age

85. Each of the following is associated with early fetal demise (abortion) EXCEPT

(a) vaccinia virus
(b) echovirus
(c) *Toxoplasma gondii*
(d) variola major

QUESTIONS 86–94

You are a solo pediatrician in a medium-small community (population 15,000) in rural Colorado. It is January, and a winter storm watch (likelihood of heavy snow in 24 hours) is in effect. You work at a Level I hospital that has the capability to stabilize but not care for ill newborns. The nearest Level II facility is 140 miles (4-hour drive) over a treacherous mountain pass, and the nearest Level III nurseries are in Denver (300 miles), which is 1 to 2 hours away by air, weather permitting. You receive a call from a family physician in a smaller town 30 miles away. He tells you that he has a patient who is in early labor at 33 or 34 weeks' gestation and asks if you would come attend the delivery "just in case there should be a problem with the baby."

86. The proper response for you to make at this point is

(a) "I'm on my way"
(b) "I'm sure you can handle it"

(c) "Bring the mother here as soon as possible"
(d) "Send the mother to Denver now"

If you answered *a* or *b*, go to question 87.
If you answered *c*, go to question 89.
If you answered *d*, go to question 90.

87. The infant is born in the small town 24 hours later, just as the storm hits. It appears to be about 34 weeks, and it weighs 1700 grams. The labor was uneventful except for some meconium-stained amniotic fluid. No analgesics or anesthetics were used during the vaginal delivery. At 20 minutes of age the infant begins to grunt audibly. The baby is placed in an incubator, and oxygen is started. Which of the following should be obtained immediately to assess the status of this infant? (Choose all that are appropriate, then go to question 88.)

(a) Blood pressure
(b) Pulse
(c) Respiratory rate
(d) Temperature
(e) Serum glucose
(f) Arterial blood gases
(g) Serum electrolytes
(h) Serum calcium
(i) Serum magnesium
(j) Complete blood count
(k) Roentgenogram of the chest

88. The blood pressure is unavailable, since there is only an adult cuff, but perfusion is poor; pulse rate is 180 per minute; respirations are 80 to 90 per minute with grunting, nasal flaring, and retractions. Temperature is 35.2°C. Serum glucose is <30 mg/dl (Dextrostix). The technician on call is trying to get in as soon as possible to do the blood gases, complete blood count, chest film, and other studies. Additional orders should include which of the following? (Choose all that are applicable and then go to answer section.)

(a) Warm the infant to 36.5°C in the incubator
(b) Umbilical arterial catheterization
(c) 10% dextrose in water, intravenously
(d) Maximum oxygen into the incubator
(e) Call for the transport team to go to the Level II center
(f) Call for the transport team to go to the Level III center

(g) Blood, urine, and cerebrospinal fluid cultures
(h) Begin penicillin and kanamycin, intravenously
(i) Sodium bicarbonate and albumin, intravenously or through the catheter
(j) Roentgenogram of the chest

89. The woman arrives at your hospital an hour later. A visiting consultant obstetrician begins a terbutaline drip, and the woman's labor stops at 3-cm dilation. You are equipped only for stabilization, but you decide to try an amniocentesis for a "shake test" of fetal maturity. The obstetrician does the amniocentesis, and the test indicates lung immaturity. More bad news is that labor begins again. Now what?

(a) Get ready for delivery
(b) Immediate transfer to Level II center
(c) Immeidate transfer to Level III in Denver

If you chose *a*, go to the answer section.
If you chose *b*, go to question 91.
If you chose *c*, go to question 90.

90. A well-to-do rancher nearby offers to fly the mother and the obstetrician to Denver. He has a pressurized Lear Jet and takes off within the hour. Unfortunately, the Denver airport closes shortly before his arrival, and he returns to the Level II facility 140 miles from your hospital. You contact your colleagues there, and they admit the patient at 4-cm dilation in active labor. (Go to question 91.)

91. The terbutaline drip at the Level II center again stops labor at 4 cm. Appropriate workup for the mother would include history, physical examination, and which of the following? (Choose all that are appropriate, then go to question 92, where all results will be given whether or not they are correct there.)

(a) Blood typing
(b) Complete blood count and urinalysis
(c) Ultrasound study of the abdomen
(d) Amniocentesis for lecithin/sphingomyelin (L/S) ratio
(e) Roentgenographic pelvimetry
(f) Vaginal culture for group B streptococci
(g) Fetal monitor

92. The patient's blood type is O + ; complete blood count and urinalysis are normal. The pelvis is adequate. Ultrasound is not working today. L/S ratio is 1.3:1, and the fetal monitor shows a normal tracing. Vaginal culture is obtained. Labor begins again 24 hours later, and the infant is delivered vaginally. He is 34 weeks and 1700 grams. At 20 minutes of age he begins grunting respirations. Which of the following should be obtained immediately to assess the status of the infant? (Choose all that are appropriate, then go to question 93, where all results will be given whether or not they are correct there.)

   (a) Blood pressure, pulse, respiratory rate, and temperature
   (b) Serum glucose
   (c) Arterial blood gases
   (d) Serum electrolytes
   (e) Serum calcium
   (f) Serum magnesium
   (g) Complete blood count
   (h) Chest roentgenogram

93.

Blood pressure	24 mm Hg
Pulse rate	180 per minute
Respirations	80 to 100 per minute with grunting and retractions
Temperature	36.4°C
Serum glucose	>45 mg/dl (Dextrostix)

Arterial blood gases (F_1O_2 = 0.40):

P_{O_2}	40 mm Hg
P_{CO_2}	50 mm HG
pH	7.19

Serum electrolytes:

Sodium	138 mEq/l
Potassium	4.9 mEq/l
Chloride	104 mEq/l
Bicarbonate	16 mEq/l
Serum calcium	9.0 mEq/l
Serum magnesium	2.0 mEq/l
Hemoglobin	15 gm/dl
Hematocrit	45%

Leukocyte count	16,000/cc mm; 70% PMNs, 30% lymphocytes
Chest roentgenogram	Complete opacification of both lung fields

Which of the following should be done now? (Choose the *one* that is appropriate, then go to question 94.)

   (a) Treat for shock, increase the inspirated oxygen, and measure blood gases
   (b) As in *a*, but also do septic work-up including lumbar puncture, and begin antibiotics
   (c) Increase oxygen, measure blood gases, and do septic work-up as in *b*
   (d) Begin continuous positive airway pressure

94. The treatment in 93 is successful. The infant's pO_2 stabilizes at 60 mm Hg, the blood pressure rises to 40 mm Hg, and the pH comes up to 7.32. Things go well until the third day when the infant has a convulsion. Laboratory evaluation (including lumbar puncture and septic work-up) is negative except for a serum sodium of 122 mEq/l. Which of the following is the most likely cause of this complication?

   (a) Forgetting to add sodium to the intravenous fluids
   (b) Inappropriate secretion of antidiuretic hormone
   (c) Sepsis
   (d) Intracranial hemorrhage
   (e) Pyroxidine deficiency
   (f) Hypocalcemia
   (g) Hypoglycemia

The infant does well. The chest film clears on the seventh day, and the oxygen requirement drops. By the eighth day, weight gain begins, and at 3 weeks of age the infant weighs 2200 grams and is discharged. The mother stops by your community to thank you for your help.

10

Special Health Problems During Adolescence

It is probably a coincidence that in the textbook this chapter on adolescence has 20 pages. While adolescence is an increasingly important area of Pediatrics, in the past it has not had its own separate chapter in the textbook (this is the second edition in which there is one). By the same token, it is fair to say that adolescents as a group are not a homogenous lot. The problems faced by younger adolescents (the 11- to 14-year-old age group) are quite different from those of older adolescents (the 15- to 20-year-old age group). This particular chapter in the textbook covers primarily the special psychosocial problems faced by adolescents in our society as well as some of the medical problems that are unique to this particular age group.

As the number of pediatric age group patients has declined in this country, the need has been perceived by many for the care of children in older age groups. Therefore, this chapter is doubly important. Perhaps by the sixth edition of this book, we will have a section on the 20- to 35-year-old age group, since by then pediatricians and those specializing in adolescent medicine may be caring for young adults.

1. The leading cause of mortality in adolescence is

    (a) violence
    (b) neoplasms
    (c) infectious disease
    (d) congential anomalies
    (e) sexually transmitted disease

2. Each of the following statements is true concerning accidents in the adolescent age group EXCEPT

    (a) Most automobile accidents involve male rather than female adolescents
    (b) Fatal accidents generally occur between 8 PM and 4 AM
    (c) Most automobile deaths among adolescents involve passengers in cars driven by adolescents
    (d) Alcohol is a major factor underlying most of these fatalities
    (e) It is not likely that increasing the legal drinking age from 18 to 21 years of age will decrease fatal automobile accidents

3. Which of the following statements is true about masked depression?

    (a) It is one of the milder forms of adolescent depression
    (b) Acting-out behavior is a hallmark
    (c) Substance abuse is not seen
    (d) Somatic symptoms are rare
    (e) Many adolescents with masked depression have psychotic breaks

4. Which of the following statements is true about adolescent suicide?

    (a) The most common method of suicide used by teenagers is ingestion of medication
    (b) The more impulsive the adolescent, the more likely the suicide is serious
    (c) Adolescents who ingest benign medications (such as antibiotics) are not as serious about committing suicide as those who consume toxic substances
    (d) Psychiatric intervention is mandatory only in serious attempts

5. Each of the following statements is true about the epidemiology of substance abuse in adolescents EXCEPT

(a) Use of heroin has leveled off at less than 1%
(b) Use of illicit drugs has declined between 1976 and 1987
(c) Marijuana remains the most widely abused substance
(d) The rates of daily use of marijuana and alcohol are similar (approximately 3 to 5%)
(e) More females than males in the adolescent age group smoke regularly

6. Which of the following statements about drug interactions is true?

(a) Estrogen contraceptives can lead to decreased alcohol metabolism
(b) Barbiturates increase the estrogen effects of contraceptives
(c) Griseofulvin has an addictive effect, thus reducing alcohol consumption
(d) Phenytoin has an Antabuse-like effect on alcohol consumption
(e) Both griseofulvin and phenytoin have an addictive effect

7. Each of the following is true of heroin use EXCEPT

(a) It produces euphoria and analgesia
(b) The intransal route is the slowest to lead to an effect
(c) Constipation and miosis are among the side effects
(d) Complications include vasodilatation, rhabdomyolosis, and cardiac arrest
(e) Withdrawal symptoms begin within 18 to 24 hours

8. Each of the following may be found in the blood of heroin addicts EXCEPT

(a) hepatitis B antibody
(b) elevated IgM
(c) elevated serum hepatic enzymes
(d) falsely negative latex fixation
(e) elevated VDRL

QUESTIONS 9–14

For each "street name," select the drug to which it refers (a–d).

9. ＿＿ Hash   (a) Jimsonweed
10. ＿＿ Locoweed   (b) Phencyclidine
11. ＿＿ Angel dust

12. ＿＿ Airplane glue   (c) Tetrahydrocannabinol
13. ＿＿ Pot   (d) Toluene
14. ＿＿ Peace pill

15. Dose-related suppression of plasma testosterone levels has been observed with chronic use of

(a) alcohol
(b) PCP
(c) marijuana
(d) airplane glue
(e) cocaine

16. An increase in daytime sleepiness and a decrease in sleep latency occurs between which of the following sexual maturity stages (SMRs)?

(a) 1–2
(b) 2–3
(c) 3–4
(d) 4–5

QUESTIONS 17–25

For each of the following symptoms or signs select the appropriate disorder (a–d).

17. ＿＿ Recurrent episodes of binge eating   (a) Anorexia nervosa
18. ＿＿ Weight loss of at least 25%   (b) Bulimia
19. ＿＿ Frequent weight fluctuations   (c) Both anorexia nervosa and bulimia
20. ＿＿ Amenorrhea
21. ＿＿ Females more affected than males   (d) None of the above
22. ＿＿ Onset at puberty
23. ＿＿ Esophagitis
24. ＿＿ Constipation
25. ＿＿ Increased susceptibility to infection

26. Which of the following best explains the reduction in pregnancy rate in the 15- to 19-year-old population?

(a) Increased use of birth control methods by boys
(b) Increased use of birth control methods by girls

(c) Increased abortion rate

(d) Decreased sexual activity by boys and girls secondary to fear of sexually transmitted diseases

27. The most commonly reported sexually transmitted disease in adolescents is

(a) gonorrhea
(b) chlamydia
(c) genital herpes
(d) condyloma acuminatum
(e) trichomonas

QUESTIONS 28–32

For each sexually transmitted disease, select the appropriate antibiotic treatment (a–f).

28. _____ Gonorrhea   (a) Acyclovir
29. _____ Herpes   (b) Metronidizole
30. _____ Condyloma   (c) Penicillin
           acuminatum   (d) Doxycycline
31. _____ Trichomonas   (e) Podophyllin
32. _____ Chlamydia   (f) Ceftriaxone

33. Menarche usually begins at which SMR?

(a) 1
(b) 2
(c) 3
(d) 4
(e) 5

34. Primary amenorrhea associated with abdominal pain, SMR 5, and a midline abdominal mass is most likely due to

(a) hyperthyroidism
(b) polycystic ovaries
(c) imperforate hymen
(d) adrenal hyperplasia
(e) chronic inflammatory bowel disease

35. Each of the following is associated with menometrorrhagia EXCEPT

(a) von Willebrand disease
(b) aspirin therapy

(c) hypothroidism
(d) Enovid therapy
(e) anovulatory cycle

36. The most common etiology for a breast mass in adolescent girls is

(a) fibroadenoma
(b) cystosarcoma phylloides
(c) abscess
(d) carcinoma

37. Each of the following disorders is more common in adolescents than younger children EXCEPT

(a) Tsetse syndrome
(b) Nongonococcal (bacterial) arthritis
(c) Osgood-Schlatter disease
(d) Idiopathic scoliosis
(e) Rubella arthralgia

38. Which of the following has been recently added to the health maintenance schedule for adolescents?

(a) dT
(b) DPT
(c) HiB
(d) MMR
(e) OPV

39. Which of the following is true?

(a) The right of a minor to consent to treatment is federally guaranteed
(b) Adolescents are generally prohibited from donating organs or blood without parental (or court) consent
(c) Emancipated minors still require parental consent for abortions
(d) The Supreme Court has upheld the minor adolescent's right to contraception

40. Which of the following is not useful as a screening procedure for all adolescents?

(a) Urinalysis
(b) Tuberculosis tests
(c) Audiometry
(d) Vision testing
(e) Blood pressure determination

11

Immunity, Allergy, and Related Diseases

In this last of the basic science review chapters in the textbook, the foundation for the host response to infection and allergens is neatly presented. Understanding the concepts in this chapter permits a more rewarding exploration of the huge area of infectious diseases that follows. Also included is an excellent review of allergy—a field that has expanded its scientific base considerably over the past decade—and a discussion of the rheumatic, autoimmune, and connective tissue diseases of childhood.

1. Which one of the following is NOT a function of T cells?

   (a) Elaboration of IgM in response to initial viral infection
   (b) Allograft rejection
   (c) Containment of mycobacterial infection
   (d) Containment of fungal infection
   (e) Containment of established viral infection

QUESTIONS 2–8

For each description, select the appropriate immunoglobulin class (a–e).

2. _____ First line of defense
3. _____ Newborn's passive immunity
4. _____ Secretory surface protection
5. _____ Effects release of agents from mast cells
6. _____ Lymphocyte receptor
7. _____ Elimination of parasites
8. _____ This and IgE are especially important to the immune status of children in underdeveloped countries

   (a) IgA
   (b) IgD
   (c) IgE
   (d) IgG
   (e) IgM

9. The presence of normal T-cell function can be assessed by which one of the following laboratory results?

   (a) Negative *Candida* skin test
   (b) Positive tuberculin skin test
   (c) Presence of large (> 10 μ diameter) lymphocytes in the peripheral smear
   (d) Roentgenogram showing retrosternal radiolucency
   (e) Diminished in vitro response to PHA (phytohemagglutinin)

10. B-cell dysfunction is confirmed by which one of the following?

    (a) Measurement of serum immunoglobulins
    (b) Response to bacteriophage φ × 174
    (c) Normal thymic shadow on roentgenogram
    (d) Protein-losing enteropathy
    (e) Reduced numbers of small (< 10 μ diameter) lymphocytes

11. An infant with eczema, thrombocytopenia, and recurrent otitis media is most likely to have which one of the following disorders?

    (a) DiGeorge syndrome
    (b) Bruton disease
    (c) Graft-versus-host disease
    (d) Wiskott-Aldrich syndrome
    (e) Nezelof syndrome

QUESTIONS 12–18

For each of the following, match the appropriate disorder (a–c).

12. _____ DiGeorge syndrome
13. _____ Ataxia-telangiectasia
14. _____ Omenn disease

    (a) T-cell deficiency

15. _____ Bruton disease
16. _____ Nezelof syndrome
17. _____ Cartilage-hair hypo-
            plasia
18. _____ Adenine deaminase
            deficiency

(b) B-cell defi-ciency
(c) Com-bined T-B cell defi-ciency

19. Which one of the following complement systems disorders can be treated with an androgen?

    (a) Systemic lupus erythematosus
    (b) Hereditary angioedema
    (c) C5 deficiency
    (d) C1q deficiency
    (e) Chronic glomerulonephritis

20. Chédiak-Higashi syndrome and chronic granulomatous disease are characterized by defects in which one of the following?

    (a) T cells
    (b) B cells
    (c) Leukocytes
    (d) Complement system
    (e) Lymph nodes

21. Which of the following is characterized by unusual susceptibility to staphylococcal infections, chronic skin lesions, and "cold" abscesses?

    (a) Chédiak-Higashi syndrome
    (b) Kartagener syndrome
    (c) Anchor disease
    (d) Schwachman syndrome
    (e) Job syndrome

22. Atopy has each of the following characteristics EXCEPT

    (a) a hereditary factor
    (b) relative but not absolute eosinophilia
    (c) predisposition to selective synthesis of IgE antibody
    (d) hyperactivity of the airway in asthma and/or hyperactivity of the skin in eczema
    (e) disturbance of the β-receptor-adenylate cyclase system

23. Which one of the following is the most sensitive test for determining hypersensitivity to specific allergens in children?

    (a) Radioallergosorbent test (RAST)
    (b) Skin testing

(c) Prausnitz-Küstner test
(d) Determination of eosinophilia
(e) Provocation testing

24. Successful treatment of allergic disorders requires each of the following EXCEPT

    (a) avoidance of allergens (environmental control)
    (b) pharmacologic therapy
    (c) judicious use of antimicrobial agents
    (d) immunotherapy (hyposensitization)
    (e) prophylaxis (e.g., breast feeding)

25. Which one of the following statements is correct?

    (a) β_2-adrenergic drugs provide bronchodilation without significantly increasing heart rate
    (b) Oral adrenergic drugs include ephedrine, isoproterenol, metaproterenol, and terbutaline
    (c) The methylxanthines (theophylline, theobromine, and caffeine) are all effective in asthma therapy
    (d) Antihistamines are effective for allergic rhinitis, but delerious in children with asthma
    (e) Cromolyn sodium in a bronchodilator that is effective in the treatment of acute asthma

26. The optimum therapeutic regimen for children requiring corticosteroids chronically is

    (a) 4 times daily
    (b) daily, between 6 and 8 AM
    (c) daily, between 4 and 6 PM
    (d) every other day, between 6 and 8 AM
    (e) every other day, between 4 and 6 PM

27. Which one of the following statements about immunotherapy (hyposensitization) is true?

    (a) Immunotherapy is indicated only in individuals suffering from asthma
    (b) Aqueous extracts of pollens, molds, and danders are manufactured under potency standards set by the United States Food and Drug Administration
    (c) There is evidence to support efficacy of immunotherapy in hay fever and in the prevention of anaphylaxis from bee stings
    (d) Injections should be continued throughout childhood
    (e) Dosage in children is reduced in proportion to weight

28. Which one of the following statements is true about allergic rhinitis?

(a) Allergic rhinitis is a predecessor of asthma in most cases

(b) Infants are most commonly affected by ragweed pollen

(c) Characteristic findings are dark circles under the eyes, allergic salute, and mouth breathing ·

(d) Nasal sympathetomimetics are effective when used daily for 1 to 2 weeks

(e) Topical (nasal) corticosteroids are ineffective

29. Each of the following statements about asthma in children is true EXCEPT

(a) The incidence is 7 to 10% of girls and 10 to 15% of boys during childhood

(b) Half of all children with asthma "grow out" of the disease by adulthood

(c) Psychologic factors are a primary cause of asthma

(d) Influenza virus and other viral agents can provoke asthmatic attacks

(e) Pathophysiologic characteristics include spasm of bronchiolar smooth muscle, edema of mucous membranes, and exudation of mucus

30. Appropriate treatment of status asthmaticus includes each of the following EXCEPT

(a) theophylline, 4 mg/kg, intravenously every 6 hours

(b) mist tent

(c) oxygen by nasal catheter

(d) intravenous fluids

(e) corticosteriods

31. Which of the following is not generally used for control of mild or moderate asthma?

(a) Cromolyn powder inhaled q.i.d.

(b) Intermittent aerosol adrenergic agents

(c) Slow-release theophylline orally daily

(d) Corticosteroids on alternate days

32. Appropriate treatment of atopic dermatitis includes each of the following EXCEPT

(a) control of environmental precipitants of itching

(b) hydration of the skin

(c) topical corticosteroids

(d) topical antibiotics if infection is present

(e) avoidance of foods clearly shown to exacerbate the disease

33. Urticaria has been definitely shown to be associated with each of the following EXCEPT

(a) infectious hepatitis

(b) cold temperatures

(c) ingestion of fish

(d) administration of penicillin

(e) psychogenic factors

34. Which one of the following statements is NOT true about anaphylaxis?

(a) Anaphylaxis in children usually results from penicillin administration or Hymenoptera stings

(b) The reaction is usually explosive and accompanied by angioedema and urticaria

(c) Death is usually related to upper airway obstruction

(d) Serious anaphylactoid reactions are common in children

(e) Immunotherapy will reduce the incidence of anaphylaxis following bee stings

QUESTIONS 35–41

A mother brings her 16-month-old infant to you with a chief complaint of "wheezing" for the last 24 hours. The infant was well until 2 days ago when he began to have a runny nose and decreased appetite. There has been fever and only an occasional cough, although the coughing has been a little worse in the past 24 hours. When wheezing began the mother became concerned and brought him to see you.

35. Which would you do now?

(a) Obtain more history (go to question 36)

(b) Perform a physical exam (go to question 37)

(c) Send the infant for laboratory and roentgenographic studies (go to question 38)

(d) Hospitalize or treat the child immediately (go to question 39)

(e) Reassure the mother and send them home

36. Choose those historical facts that are pertinent to the management of this child. (Choose as many as are appropriate, then go to question 37)

(a) Has anyone else been ill at home?

(b) Has he ever wheezed before?

(c) Is there a family history of allergy or asthma?

(d) What did the rhinorrhea look like?

(e) Was the rhinorrhea bilateral or unilateral?

(f) Has he aspirated or choked on any food?

(g) Has he had any drugs?

(h) Is he being given vitamins?

(i) Hs he turned blue?

(j) Has he stopped breathing at any time?

(k) Are his immunizations up to date?

(l) Is he allergic to anything?

37. Physical examination reveals a well-developed, well-hydrated, well-nourished infant in moderate respiratory distress. Temperature is 37.7°C. Respirations are 60 to 70 per minute with retractions and audible expiratory wheezing. Pulse is 150 per minute, and blood pressure is 70 mm Hg systolic by palpation. Moderate clear rhinorrhea and mild perioral cyanosis are noted. There are bilateral generalized expiratory wheezes with occasional intermittent rales throughout both lung fields. The liver is palpable 3 cm below the right costal margin, and the spleen tip is palpable. What would you do now?

(a) Reassure the mother and send them home

(b) Start antibiotics and see the child again in 24 hours

(c) Obtain laboratory and roentgenographic studies (go to question 38.)

(d) Hospitalize or treat the child immediately (go to question 41)

38. Which of the following would you order? (Choose as many as are appropriate, then go to question 39.)

(a) Complete blood count
(b) Urinalysis
(c) Serum electrolytes
(d) Blood urea nitrogen
(e) Serum calcium
(f) Arterial blood gases
(g) Nose culture
(h) Throat culture
(i) Blood culture
(j) Urine culture
(k) Cerebrospinal fluid culture
(l) Pulmonary function testing
(m) Posteroanterior and lateral roentgenograms of chest
(n) Inspiratory-expiratory chest films
(o) Viral cultures and serology

39. The laboratory results for question 38 are listed, regardless of whether they were considered pertinent.

Hematocrit	37%
Hemoglobin	12.2 gm/dl
Leukocyte count	8200/cu mm; 22% PMNs, 75% lymphocytes, 1% monocytes, 2% eosinophils
Urinalysis	Specific gravity 1.015; pH 6.0; protein, glucose and ketones negative; microscopic negative

Serum electrolytes:

Sodium	141 mEq/l
Potassium	4.5 mEq/l
Chloride	101 mEq/l
Bicarbonate	18 mEq/l
Blood urea nitrogen	10 mg/dl
Serum calcium	4.4 mEq/l

Arterial blood studies:

P_{O_2}	60 mm Hg
P_{CO_2}	32 mm Hg
pH	7.36
Nose culture	Pending
Throat culture	Pending
Blood culture	Pending
Urine culture	Pending
Cerebrospinal fluid culture	Pending
Pulmonary function testing	Scheduled
PA and lateral chest films	Hyperexpansion of lung fields; diffuse interstitial patchy infiltrates
Inspiratory-expiratory film	Negative
Viral cultures and serology	Pending

Based on the information you have so far, you would now

(a) Reassure the mother and send them home

(b) Hospitalize or treat the child immediately (go to question 36)

40. Whether in the hospital or in the office, list sequentially the therapies you would attempt for this child.

_____ (a) Aminophylline, 4 mg/kg intravenously

_____ (b) 1:1000 aqueous epinephrine, 0.01 ml/kg subcutaneously, × 3 if necessary

_____ (c) Aminophylline, 5 mg/kg orally

_____ (d) Nasal oxygen at 2 to 3 liters/minute

_____ (e) Albuterol, 0.15 mg/kg, diluted and inhaled by nebulizer

_____ (f) Prednisone, 2 mg/kg orally

_____ (g) Cromolyn sodium inhaler, 2 times daily

41. The most likely diagnosis in this infant is

(a) viral pneumonia
(b) mycoplasma pneumonia
(c) bacterial pneumonia
(d) asthma
(e) bronchiolitis

42. Each of the following statements is true of serum sickness in children EXCEPT

(a) It is an immune complex disease
(b) Glomerulonephritis is a major finding
(c) Symptoms begin 7 to 12 days after injection of foreign material
(d) Serum complement (C3, C4) is sometimes depressed on day 10
(e) Treatment with aspirin and antihistamines or steroids is effective in severe cases

43. Histocompatability antigen HLA B27 is associated with which one of the following diseases?

(a) Ankylosing spondylitis
(b) Juvenile rheumatoid arthritis (Still disease)
(c) Pauciarticular type I juvenile rheumatoid arthritis (JRA)
(d) Polyarticular JRA
(e) Chronic active hepatitis

44. Which of the following is the drug of choice for the initial treatment of JRA?

(a) Corticosteroids, orally
(b) Corticosteroids, intrasynovially
(c) Salicylates, orally
(d) Gold, intramuscularly
(e) Acetaminophen, orally

45. Each of the following statements about lupus erythematosus is true EXCEPT

(a) Sex ratio of girls to boys after puberty is 8:1
(b) Antinuclear antibodies are present in active cases
(c) Drugs including steroids, antimalarials, and antimetabolites may be therapeutically used
(d) Renal involvement (nephritis) is common
(e) 90% of children survive 5 years

46. A child has abdominal pain, low-grade fever, arthritis, microscopic hematuria, and a purpuric rash only on the lower extremeties. Which of the following is the most likely diagnosis?

(a) Meningococcemia
(b) Varicella
(c) Schönlein-Henoch vasculitis
(d) Post-streptococcal glomerulonephritis
(e) Infectious mononucleosis

47. High fever, conjunctivitis, stomatitis, palmar erythema and desquamation of the digits, significant lymphadenopathy, and carditis are characteristics of

(a) polyarteritis nodosa
(b) Good pasture syndrome
(c) erythema nodosum
(d) mucocutaneous lymph node syndrome (Kawasaki disease)
(e) Wegener granulomatosis

48. Which of the following therapies may prevent the coronary manifestations of Kawasaki disease?

(a) Aspirin
(b) Azothiaprine
(c) Cyclophosphamide
(d) Intravenous gamma globulin
(e) Methotrexate

49. Corticosteroids are effective in the treatment of which of the following?

(a) Scleroderma
(b) Dermatomyositis
(c) Erythema nodosum
(d) Lyme disease (erythema chronicum migrans)
(e) none of the above

QUESTIONS 50–54

From the accompanying list (a–j), identify the five major manifestations of rheumatic fever (modified Jones criteria). Assume evidence of streptococcal infection.

50. _____ (a) Fever
51. _____ (b) Carditis
52. _____ (c) Arthralgia
53. _____ (d) Polyarthritis
54. _____ (e) Chorea

(f) Elevated erythrocyte sedimentation rate
(g) Subcutaneous nodules
(h) Erythema marginatum
(i) Erythema multiforme
(j) Elevated ASO tier

55. Factors associated with the decline in incidence of rheumatic fever prior to the mid-1980s include each of the following EXCEPT

(a) use of throat cultures for pharyngitis
(b) use of antimicrobials, especially penicillin
(c) development of comprehensive health care clinics in inner city neighborhoods
(d) passage of Medicaid legislation
(e) use of vaccines (anti-streptococcal)

12

Infectious Diseases

This is a monumental chapter. It comprehensively reviews infectious diseases of children, including syndromes and specific etiologic entities, as well as much background material in laboratory diagnosis. The format of this review will be specific questions relating to the text material and more than the usual number of case-oriented management problems.

1. Which one of the following statements is true about fever of unknown origin (FUO) in children?

    (a) Most children with FUO are eventually found to have neoplastic disease
    (b) Infections and collagen-vascular etiologies predominate
    (c) True FUO occurs when a fever is undiagnosed after 1 week
    (d) Acetaminophen is effective treatment for most cases of FUO
    (e) Bacterial endotoxins are the most common cause of FUO

QUESTIONS 2–5

For each organism, select the appropriate diagnostic technique (a–d).

2. _____ Gonococ-   (a) Blood agar
     cus   (b) Thayer-Martin
3. _____ Rubella   medium
     virus   (c) Giemsa stain
4. _____ Strepto-   (d) Hemagglutination
     coccus   inhibition
5. _____ Chlamy-
     dia

6. Each of the following organisms elaborates a toxin which causes diarrhea EXCEPT

    (a) *Yersinia enterocolitica*
    (b) *Vibrio cholera*
    (c) *Staphylococcus aureus*
    (d) *Shigella dysenteriae*
    (e) Enterotoxigenic *Escherichia coli*

7. Aseptic meningitis in the United States has as its etiologic agent which of the following in 85% of cases?

    (a) Retroviruses
    (b) Arboviruses
    (c) Mumps virus
    (d) Enteroviruses
    (e) Herpes simplex

8. The most common etiology for bacterial meningitis in 3-year-olds is

    (a) *Neisseria meningiditis*
    (b) *Streptococcus pneumoniae*
    (c) *Staphylococcus aureus*
    (d) *Haemophilus influenza* type B
    (e) *Mycobacterium tuberculosis*

QUESTIONS 9–14

For each of the following situations noted in a 2-year-old child, select the appropriate diagnosis (a–d).

9. _____ Limping   (a) Osteomyelitis
10. _____ Sickle-cell (b) Septic arthritis
     disease   (c) Both osteomyeli-
     and sal-   tis and septic ar-
     monella   thritis
     isolate   (d) None of the
11. _____ *Staphylo-*   above
     coccus au-
     reus most
     common
12. _____ *Haemo-*
     philus
     most com-
     mon
13. _____ Antibiotic
     therapy
     for 7 to 10
     days
14. _____ Surgical
     drainage
     if no re-
     sponse in
     48 hours

15. Which of the following statements concerning group A streptococcal infection is true?

    (a) Pharyngitis is most common in infants
    (b) Skin infection is more common than pharyngitis in tropical climates
    (c) Most infections occur in the summer
    (d) The carrier state does *not* confer immunity
    (e) Serious sequelae occur in approximately 10% of cases

16. Each of the following may be attributed to streptococcal infection EXCEPT

    (a) low-grade fever, thin watery rhinorrhea, and cervical adenopathy in a 9-month-old child
    (b) fever, abdominal pain, and tonsillitis in a 6-year-old child
    (c) fever, rash, and pharyngitis in a 10-year-old child
    (d) cellulitis, lymphangitis, and lymphadenitis in a 3-year-old child
    (e) bullous pyoderma in a newborn

17. Confirmation of the diagnosis of streptococcal infection best relies on which one of the following?

    (a) Clinical history
    (b) Physical findings
    (c) Isolation of the organism
    (d) Increase in antistreptolysin O (ASO) titer (fourfold or more)
    (e) Epidemiologic data

18. Which one of the following treatment regimens is NOT satisfactory for streptococcal infection?

    (a) Erythromycin, 40 mg/kg, orally daily
    (b) Penicillin G, 800,000 units, orally daily in 4 divided doses for 10 days
    (c) Benzathine penicillin, 1.2 million units, intramuscularly
    (d) Tetracycline, 250 mg, orally 4 times daily (if child is older than 7 years)
    (e) Lincomycin, 40 mg/kg, orally daily

19. Each of the following statements about *Staphylococcus aureus* is true EXCEPT

    (a) It can cause tonsillopharyngitis
    (b) It can cause scarlet fever by elaboration of an erythrogenic toxin

    (c) It is a common cause of acute bacterial endocarditis
    (d) Certain strains elaborate an enterotoxin that is a common cause of food poisoning
    (e) It is the etiologic agent of Ritter disease and Lyell disease

20. Which statement is correct concerning the prevention or treatment of staphylococcal infections?

    (a) The best prevention is handwashing
    (b) Specific penicillinase-resistant antibiotics will cure most staphylococcal abscesses
    (c) Clindamycin is effective for treating meningitis in children who are allergic to penicillin
    (d) Specific vaccines are available for prevention of staphylococcal infections
    (e) Prophylactic penicillin is effective in diminishing cord colonization

21. Which of the following statements is true about pneumococcal diseases?

    (a) Incidence is highest in school-age children
    (b) Pneumococci must invade to produce disease
    (c) Epidemics generally occur in the winter
    (d) Pneumococcal infection occurs independently of viral infection
    (e) Pneumococcal vaccines are effective in infants

22. The antibiotic of choice for most proven pneumococcal infection is

    (a) penicillin
    (b) tetracycline
    (c) a sulfonamide
    (d) streptomycin
    (e) vancomycin

23. Each of the following statements concerning infection due to *Haemophilus influenzae* is true EXCEPT

    (a) The encapsulated strains of *H. influenzae* are associated with pathogenicity and severe infections
    (b) Unencapsulated (nontypable) strains have been implicated in otitis media
    (c) *H. influenzae* is the leading cause of meningitis in the first 4 years of life

(d) Infection in infants can be prevented by the use of a polysaccharide vaccine

(e) Type b is a common cause of epiglottitis and meningitis

24. Poor prognostic signs for patients with meningococcal infection include all of the following EXCEPT

(a) meningitis
(b) hypotension
(c) leukopenia
(d) low erythrocyte sedimentation rate
(e) thrombocytopenia

25. Which of the following is the antibiotic of choice for patients with documented meningococcemia?

(a) Penicillin V (phenoxymethyl penicillin)
(b) Penicillin G
(c) Erythromycin
(d) Ampicillin
(e) Oxacillin

26. Which statement about gonococcal infection is NOT true?

(a) It is the most commonly reported infectious disease in the United States
(b) It is often asymptomatic
(c) A presumptive diagnosis in both men and women can be obtained by Gram stain of urethral discharge
(d) Ophthalmologic infection in neonates can be prevented by the administration of 1% silver nitrate solution
(e) The number of cases reported in school-aged children is increasing

27. Which one of the following statements regarding diphtheria is true?

(a) The incidence is highest in the spring and summer
(b) It occurs primarily in unimmunized individuals
(c) The incubation period is 1 to 2 weeks
(d) The incidence has remained unchanged over the past 30 years despite the use of toxoid
(e) The incidence is highest in health personnel

28. Each of the following statements about diphtheria is true EXCEPT

(a) Pathologic disease is caused by invasion of the bacterium into tissue

(b) Nasal diphtheria is most common in infants
(c) Treatment should *not* await laboratory confirmation of the disease
(d) Death in laryngeal diphtheria occurs from obstruction of airway rather than toxigenic effects on other organs
(e) Patients who recover should be immunized with toxoid because of lack of antibody response to the toxin

29. Which of the following is most appropriate for treating diphtheria?

(a) Penicillin, 600,000 units, intramuscularly daily
(b) Penicillin as in *a*, plus antitoxin
(c) Penicillin as in *a*, plus diphtheria toxoid
(d) Penicillin as in *a*, plus antitoxin and diphtheria toxoid
(e) Antitoxin and diphtheria toxoid without penicillin

30. Pertussis is best treated with which of the following?

(a) Erythromycin
(b) Erythromycin and pertussis immune globulin
(c) Penicillin
(d) Penicillin and pertussis immune globulin
(e) Pertussis immune globulin

31. Which of the following statements regarding infections caused by enteropathogenic *Escherichia coli* in infants is true?

(a) They are characterized by many leukocytes and erythrocytes in the stools
(b) They respond well to kaolin or diphenoxylate and atropine (Lomotil)
(c) Mortality in infants is usually the result of dehydration
(d) They are primarily water-borne
(e) They lead to hepatic abscesses

32. Each one of the following conditions increases susceptibility to infection with salmonellae EXCEPT

(a) sickle-cell anemia
(b) systemic lupus erythematosus
(c) gastric hyperacidity and ulcer disease
(d) malaria
(e) Hodgkin disease

33. Each of the following statements about typhoid fever is true EXCEPT

(a) The carrier state can be eradicated by cholecystectomy in 80% of cases
(b) Typhoid vaccine is highly effective in eliminating disease from endemic areas
(c) Chloramphenicol and ampicillin are the antibiotics of choice
(d) Intestinal perforation and severe hemorrhage are complications in the second stage of the illness
(e) Peripheral leukocyte counts are generally low unless abscesses are present

34. Which one of the following is true about shigellosis?

(a) Neurologic complications occur in about 40% of patients
(b) Animal reservoirs include poultry and shellfish
(c) Neomycin, orally, is the antibiotic of choice
(d) Bacteremia is common
(e) The disease is rare in institutions for the retarded

35. Each of the following statements about *Pseudomonas aeruginosa* is true EXCEPT

(a) It lives primarily in soil and water
(b) The infection is opportunistic
(c) Pneumonia and septicemia are common in children with cystic fibrosis
(d) A vaccine and hyperimmune globulin are effective for treating burn patients
(e) It is a gram-negative rod

QUESTIONS 36–39

For each organism, select its reservoir or vector (a–e)

36. _____ *Brucella abortus*   (a) Fleas
37. _____ *Brucella melitensis*   (b) Rabbits
(c) Cows
38. _____ *Yersinia pestis*   (d) Goats
(e) Mosquitos
39. _____ *Francisella tularensis*

40. Each of the following is a type of tularemia EXCEPT

(a) typhoidal
(b) oculoglandular
(c) oropharyngeal
(d) meningitis
(e) ulceroglandular

41. Which of the following antibiotics is the treatment of choice for plague, for tularemia, and in combination with tetracycline, for recurrent brucellosis?

(a) Penicillin
(b) Sulfacetamide
(c) Streptomycin
(d) Erythromycin
(e) Ampicillin

42. The symptoms and clinical presentation of infection with *Listeria* in newborns are most similar to those of which of the following illnesses?

(a) Group A streptococcal infection
(b) Group B streptococcal infection
(c) *Pseudomonas aeruginosa* infection
(d) *Haemophilus influenzae* infection
(e) Meningococcus infection

43. Each of the following forms of anthrax has been described EXCEPT

(a) meningeal
(b) gastrointestinal
(c) pulmonary
(d) cutaneous
(e) hepatic

44. Which one of the following statements is accurate with respect to tetanus?

(a) The case fatality rate has declined dramatically during the past 20 years
(b) Tetanolysin, an exotoxin, is responsible for the clinical symptoms
(c) Most newborns with tetanus are born to unimmunized mothers in unsterile conditions
(d) Antitoxin will reverse the effects of tissue-bound toxin
(e) The disease provides lifelong immunity

45. A 14-year-old farmer's son comes to the emergency room 26 hours after he tripped over a barbed wire fence and fell into a pile of cow manure, sustaining a puncture wound of the right hand. His parents tell you that he had "one, maybe two, baby shots" but none in recent memory. Appropriate treatment for this young man would include all of the following EXCEPT

(a) thorough washing and débridement of the wound
(b) administration of penicillin
(c) administration of tetanus immune globulin
(d) administration of tetanus toxoid and diphtheria toxoid (Td)
(e) quarantine

46. Which statement is true about botulism?

(a) Most cases are food related with ingestion of toxin
(b) Boiling for 10 minutes will kill the spores of *Clostridium*
(c) Antibiotics have little place in its treatment
(d) Newborns are affected more severely than older children and adults
(e) A vaccine is available for high-risk laboratory personnel

47. Each of the following is a clue to anaerobic infection EXCEPT

(a) no growth on routine cultures
(b) positive Gram stain and no growth in aerobic cultures
(c) characteristic colony formation in cultures held in reduced (10 to 15%) oxygen
(d) production of gas and foul odor in vivo or in vitro
(e) growth in thioglycolate broth

48. Penicillin is effective against each of the following EXCEPT

(a) *Bacteroides fragilis*
(b) *Clostridium tetani*
(c) Fusobacteria
(d) *Clostridium botulinum*
(e) *Bacillus subtilis*

QUESTIONS 49–54

For each "opportunity," select the most likely cause of infection (a–e).

49. _____ Burns
50. _____ Urethral catheters

(a) *Staphylococcus epidermidis*
(b) *Escherichia coli*

51. _____ Ventriculoperitoneal shunts
52. _____ Inhalation therapy equipment
53. _____ Chronic granulomatous disease
54. _____ Dermal sinus tracts

(c) *Pseudomonas aeruginosa*
(d) *Serratia marcescens*
(e) *Staphylococcus aureus*

QUESTIONS 55–59

Match the symptomatology in the left column with the likely agent on the right (a–d).

55. _____ Draining, infected dog bite
56. _____ Watery, then bloody diarrhea
57. _____ Pneumonia, normal host
58. _____ Fever, myalgias, headache
59. _____ Subcutaneous "woody" mass

(a) *Legionella pneumophila*
(b) *Pasteurella multocida*
(c) *Campylobacter fetus*
(d) *Actinomyces*

60. Which of the following statements about tuberculosis is true?

(a) BCG is effective and should be used routinely in newborns in the United States
(b) Acquisition of measles (rubeola) will exacerbate tuberculosis in children
(c) Sputum cultures are the most effective method to diagnose tuberculosis in infants
(d) Chemotherapy is effective in preventing tuberculosis
(e) Miliary tuberculosis most commonly occurs in adolescents

61. Which of the following is most appropriate for treatment of an infant with miliary tuberculosis or tuberculosis meningitis?

    (a) Isoniazid (INH) and para-aminosalicyclic acid (PAS)
    (b) INH, rifampin, and streptomycin
    (c) Rifampin and streptomycin
    (d) INH and ethionamide
    (e) Corticosteroids and PAS

62. Which of the following is the most likely congenital cause of rash, severe rhinorrhea, and pseudoparalysis of the limbs in a 1-month-old infant?

    (a) Rubella
    (b) Tuberculosis
    (c) Leprosy
    (d) Syphilis
    (e) Toxoplasmosis

63. Each of the following is caused by treponema EXCEPT

    (a) syphilis
    (b) bejel
    (c) yaws
    (d) pinta
    (e) Weil disease

64. Pneumonia has been etiologically implicated in each of the following EXCEPT

    (a) mycoplasmas
    (b) chlamydia
    (c) mycobacteria
    (d) plasmodia
    (e) rickettsiae

65. Each of the following statements about measles is true EXCEPT

    (a) Koplik spots are pathognomonic
    (b) The peak contagiousness occurs during the rash, which lasts 7 to 10 days
    (c) Complications include pneumonia, otitis media, and encephalitis
    (d) Both active and passive immunization will prevent the disease
    (e) The rate of encephalitis following immunization is 1000 times less than that following natural disease

66. Which of the following statements is true of rubella?

    (a) It has a shorter incubation period than measles

    (b) It is associated with thrombocytopenia and arthritis
    (c) It is associated with nerve deafness
    (d) It has a rash that appears following lysis of fever
    (e) It occurs in 2- to 4-year epidemics

67. A 7-month-old infant suddenly develops a fever of 40.0°C. No other symptoms are present, and no significant physical findings are found other than mild coryza and posterior cervical adenopathy. The child looks quite well. Which one of the following statements best describes the diagnostic factors to be considered in this case?

    (a) A rash appearing within 24 hours of onset of fever would make roseola a likely diagnosis
    (b) Pneumococcal fever should be excluded by complete blood count and/or blood cultures
    (c) The fever could be the prodrome of rubella
    (d) If the fever persists for 3 days and then abruptly falls, with onset of rash at that time, erythema infectiosum would be the likely diagnosis
    (e) Scarlet fever is likely, since it is a disease of 6- to 18-month-old infants

68. Which of the following is true about herpesvirus infections?

    (a) Most neonatal herpes is caused by type 1 virus
    (b) Repeated smallpox immunization will eliminate recurrent stomatitis
    (c) Primary infection in infants usually leads to fever of 4 to 9 days' duration
    (d) Type 2 herpesvirus can be treated effectively with hyperimmune gamma globulin
    (e) Herpesvirus causes epidemic keratoconjunctivitis

69. Which of the following statements is true of varicella?

    (a) Crusts are infectious
    (b) Varicella virus and zoster virus are the same agent
    (c) The lesions are clinically easily distinguished from those of herpes simplex
    (d) The vaccine is indicated for routine use in children of school age
    (e) Zoster immune globulin is of *no* proven value in children

70. Which of the following statements about cytomegalovirus (CMV) infection is true?

(a) 90% of newborns with congenital infection are symptomatic
(b) The virus is highly contagious
(c) Acquired infection is easily confused with infectious mononucleosis
(d) A CMV vaccine is available for patients who are immunosuppressed
(e) Infection occurs by the oral route only

71. Each of the following statements is true about infectious mononucleosis EXCEPT

(a) Lymphocytes infected with Epstein-Barr (EB) virus will grow perpetually in tissue culture
(b) The less affluent the population, the more likely the presence of antibody to EB virus
(c) The classic findings include pharyngitis, posterior cervical lymphadenopathy, and hepatosplenomegaly
(d) Rashes occur in 80% of patients who have infectious mononucleosis and who are receiving ampicillin
(e) Corticosteroids are indicated for most cases

72. Which of the following is true about mumps?

(a) The mumps skin test is a reliable indicator of immunity
(b) The incubation period is 7 to 10 days
(c) Meningoencephalitis can precede, occur simultaneously with, or follow parotitis
(d) Salivary gland involvement is limited to the parotids
(e) Infertility is common following mumps orchitis

73. Complications of influenza virus infection include each of the following EXCEPT

(a) Reye syndrome
(b) glossitis
(c) otitis media
(d) sinusitis
(e) pneumonia

74. Viral "croup" can be caused by each of the following EXCEPT

(a) measles virus
(b) influenza A/Hong Kong/68
(c) influenza A/Texas/77

(d) parainfluenza type 2
(e) parainfluenza type 4

75. Hemorrhagic cystitis, conjunctivitis, pneumonia, and diarrhea have all been etiologically linked to which one of the following?

(a) Respiratory syncytial virus
(b) Adenovirus
(c) Rhinovirus
(d) Herpesvirus
(e) Parainfluenza virus

76. Which of the following statements is true about respiratory syncytial virus (RSV) infection?

(a) Apnea and periodic breathing may be presenting symptoms
(b) The older the child is at time of first infection, the more severe the disease
(c) The primary disease form is pneumonia
(d) Inactivated RSV vaccines are effective but not yet licensed
(e) Transplacental antibody is protective for the first 3 to 6 months of life

77. Which statement is NOT true about hepatitis?

(a) Hepatitis A (infectious hepatitis) is highly contagious by the fecal-oral route
(b) Hepatitis B (serum hepatitis) is transmitted only by the parenteral route
(c) Most hepatitis A infections in children are subclinical
(d) Arthralgia and skin eruptions are seen in hepatitis B infection
(e) Acute fulminant hepatitis more often follows hepatitis A than hepatitis B

78. Each of the following is a picornavirus EXCEPT

(a) poliovirus, type II
(b) coxsackievirus A, type 16
(c) echovirus, type 9
(d) attenuated (Sabin strain) poliovirus, type III
(e) adenovirus, type 8

79. A 2-year-old child living in New York City is bitten by a dog. After cleaning and washing the wound, which of the following should be done next?

(a) Find the dog and observe it

(b) Begin rabies hyperimmune globulin
(c) Vaccinate the child with duck embryo vaccine
(d) Give both immune globulin and vaccine

QUESTIONS 80–87

For each disease, select the appropriate vector (a–e).

80. _____ Colorado tick fever   (a) Mosquitoes
81. _____ Rocky Mountain spotted fever   (b) Fleas   (c) Ticks   (d) Lice   (e) Mites
82. _____ Yellow fever
83. _____ Epidemic typhus
84. _____ Endemic typhus
85. _____ Scrub typhus
86. _____ Dengue fever
87. _____ Rickettsialpox

---

88. Mycotic infections include each of the following EXCEPT

(a) atypical mycobacterial infection
(b) blastomycosis
(c) cryptococcosis
(d) histoplasmosis
(e) aspergillosis

89. Each of the following statements regarding coccidioidomycosis is true EXCEPT

(a) It is usually a self-limited, benign fungal infection of man
(b) Pulmonary cavitation occasionally occurs
(c) Dissemination rarely occurs
(d) It is primarily a disease of residents of the San Joaquin Valley in California and of the desert Southwest
(e) A vaccine is available for prevention of the disease in children

QUESTIONS 90–92

A 10-year-old boy is brought to your New York City office with a 2-week history of fever and malaise. No other family members or friends are ill, and he has had no known exposure to tuberculosis. His parents, both of whom are physicians, are moderately paranoid and convinced that he has leukemia. On physical examination the boy appears tired and ill; there is mild pallor. The chest is clear. The spleen is enlarged and palpable 3 cm below the left costal margin. The examination is otherwise unremarkable.

90. Which additional historical facts would you want to ascertain? (Choose as many as are relevant, then go to question 91, where all of the answers will be reported, whether or not they are correct there.)

(a) Presence of nausea, vomiting, or diarrhea
(b) Upper respiratory symptoms, cough, coryza, etc.
(c) Recent travel from New York
(d) Immunization history
(e) Past history of childhood diseases, mononucleosis, or other communicable illnesses
(f) Family history of cancer or other illnesses
(g) Review of systems
(h) Recent injection of or exposure to toxins
(i) Medications

91. On further questioning, you find that the patient has had no gastrointestinal or respiratory symptoms, and that apart from 2 weeks last month with his grandparents on a farm in central Missouri, he has not been out of the city. His immunizations are all up to date. He had varicella 5 years ago, but there is no history of mononucleosis. A paternal grandmother died of cancer of the colon at age 97; there are five deaths from heart disease in the last three generations, all at age 70 to 80. Review of systems is negative, and he has had no exposure to toxins other than in the course of breathing city air. He is taking no medications. Which of the following laboratory studies would you order initially? (Choose all that are appropriate, then go to question 92.)

(a) Complete blood count
(b) Urinalysis
(c) Sinus films
(d) Chest films

(e) Upper gastrointestinal series
(f) Barium enema
(g) Intravenous urogram
(h) Erythrocyte sedimentation rate
(i) Acute serum for viral studies
(j) Monospot test
(k) Proteus OX-2 and OX-19 antibodies
(l) Brucella and tularemia antibodies
(m) Tuberculin skin test (PPD), intermediate strength)
(n) Histoplasmin skin test
(o) Atypical mycobacteria skin tests
(p) Coccidioidin skin test
(q) Blastomyces skin test

92. Laboratory studies (all results reported, whether or not correct in question 91).

Hematocrit	34%
Hemoglobin	11.0 gm/dl
Leukocyte count	5500/cu mm; 25% PMNs, 70% lymphocytes, 3% monocytes, 2% eosinophils
Erythrocyte sedimentation rate	20 mm/hour
Monospot test	Negative
Viral studies	Acute serum drawn and saved
Skin tests:	Results at 48 hours:
Tuberculin	Negative
Histoplasmin	20 mm induration
Atypical mycobacteria	Negative
Coccidioidin	Negative
Blastomyces	Negative
Serology:	
Brucella agglutinins	1:10
Tularemia agglutinins	1:20
Proteus (OX-2, OX-19)	1:10, 1:10
Sinus films	Negative
Chest films	Enlarged mediastinal lymph nodes
Upper GI series	Negative
Barium enema	Negative
Intravenous urogram	Negative

The most appropriate *initial* therapy for this patient would be

(a) penicillin, 400,000 units, intravenously

(b) amphotericin B, 0.1 mg/kg, intravenously daily
(c) sulfonamides (Triple Sulfa), 150 mg/kg, orally daily
(d) griseofulvin 5 mg, orally 4 times daily
(e) no treatment indicated

93. Each of the following has been associated with ascaris infection in humans EXCEPT

(a) asthma
(b) urticaria
(c) Löeffler-like syndrome
(d) anemia
(e) intussusception

94. A 3-year-old child has a low-grade fever, cough, and a leukocyte count of 90,000/cu mm with 90% eosinophils. The most likely cause is

(a) *Ascaris lumbricoides*
(b) *Enterobius vermicularis*
(c) *Toxocara canis*
(d) *Trichuris trichiura*
(e) *Ancylostoma duodenale*

95. Which one of the following parasites does NOT infect man by the percutaneous route?

(a) Strongyloides
(b) Ancylostoma
(c) Echinococcus
(d) Schistosoma
(e) Necator

96. Specific antivenin is available for the treatment of which one of the following?

(a) Myiasis
(b) Tick paralysis
(c) Black widow spider bite
(d) Honeybee bite
(e) Scabies

97. Each of the following diseases is caused by a protozoan EXCEPT

(a) paragonimiasis
(b) malaria
(c) leishmaniasis
(d) giardiasis
(e) Chagas disease

98. Which statement is true about toxoplasmosis?

(a) The second child born to a mother whose first child had congenital tox-

oplasmosis is at higher risk for being affected than the population
(b) Maternal infection in the first trimester is *not* as dangerous to the fetus as a third-trimester infection
(c) Acquired toxoplasmosis in pregnant women is usually symptomatic
(d) Most maternal infections do not lead to congenital infection
(e) Toxoplasmosis is a common cause of cerebral palsy

99. A protozoan causing infection and intestinal symptoms in mountain resorts in the United States is

(a) *Balantidium coli*
(b) *Giardia lamblia*
(c) *Entamoeba histolytica*
(d) *Toxoplasma gondii*
(e) *Trichomonas vaginalis*

QUESTIONS 100–105

It is 1 AM and the telephone rings in your home. The answering service tells you that Mrs. Jackson is on the line and would like to talk with you about her son Casper. You walk to another telephone in the house trying hard to wake up in order to have a lucid conversation, and trying to remember something about Casper. The maneuver is successful, and as you reach the kitchen telephone, you remember that Casper is 9 months old and that you last saw him a week ago for a "well child" check-up. At that time you administered live attenuated measles vaccine. Previously, Casper had received three DPT and two OPV shots. Mrs. Jackson, you remember, seems to be a conscientious mother, not prone to anxiety, and this is the first time she has called at night. Your conversation elicits the following: Casper was well until 2 days ago when he developed a runny nose and cough. At about 8 o'clock tonight he suddenly developed a temperature of 39.0°C and began crying. He would not sleep, and only occasionally nursed on the left breast. He refused the right breast. She had given him 0.3 ml of acetaminophen without success at 10 PM, and when it appeared that things were not improving she called.

100. At this point you should

(a) reassure Mrs. Jackson that the fever is probably a reaction to the measles

vaccine and that Casper will be fine in a few days.
(b) call a prescription for an antibiotic (go to question 101)
(c) meet Mrs. Jackson and Casper in the emergency room of the hospital (go to question 103)
(d) Suggest doubling the dose of acetaminophen to 0.6 ml and also give one baby aspirin and call back in the morning (go to question 102)

101. Appropriate antibiotics would include which of the following?

(a) Penicillin G
(b) Penicillin V
(c) Penicillin V and sulfonamides (Triple Sulfa)
(d) Ampicillin
(e) Erythromycin and sulfonamides

102. Mrs. Jackson calls back at 3 AM saying that the fever is down a little, but Casper is more irritable than before, and you sense that she is too. Meet her in the emergency room in question 103.

103. On arrival in the emergency room you find an irritable baby with a temperature of 39.0°C and the following physical findings: soft, flat fontanelle, cerumen-packed ear canals, 4+ bubbly rhinorrhea, mildly injected pharynx, and slightly increased posterior cervical lymph nodes. No Koplik spots are seen. The rest of the physical exam is unremarkable. Which of the following would you do now? (Choose as many as are appropriate.)

(a) Try to remove the cerumen (go to question 104)
(b) Reassure Mrs. Jackson that Casper has only an upper respiratory infection and you will see him again in a few days if he does not improve; prescribe a wax softener (go to question 104)
(c) Begin an antibiotic (go to question 101) and send them home
(d) Get a complete blood count and roentgenogram of the chest (go to question 104)

104. The most likely diagnosis in this case is

(a) measles
(b) measles vaccine reaction

(c) upper respiratory infection
(d) otitis media in the left ear
(e) pneumonia

105. Casper's next follow-up appointment(s) should be

(a) 2 weeks later
(b) 2 weeks and 6 months later
(c) 3 months later
(d) 3 months and 6 months later
(e) 6 months later

106. Three months after the preceding episode, in the middle of winter, you get another 1 AM call from Mrs. Jackson. This time she tells you that Casper has a croupy cough. You elicit the further history that he has had an upper respiratory infection for 2 days (as has the whole family), and he suddenly awoke with a fever of 39.0°C, a croupy cough, and restlessness. He is not drooling and will drink some fluids. You tell Mrs. Jackson to meet you in the emergency room, and when you get there you find Casper croupy and very restless. Which of the following is the most appropriate course of action?

(a) Order a complete blood count and roentgenogram of the chest
(b) Visualize the epiglottis and intubate if it is enlarged
(c) Oxygenate, visualize the epiglottis, and intubate if it is enlarged; admit and observe
(d) Admit Casper to the hospital and give humidified oxygen nasally
(e) Admit to the hospital for observation and begin antibiotics and steroids

107. The most likely diagnosis at this time is

(a) *Hemophilus influenzae* epiglottitis
(b) viral croup
(c) allergic or "spasmodic" croup
(d) diphtheria
(e) foreign body in the larynx

QUESTIONS 108–113

For each of the following pairs of serologic test results, match the appropriate diagnosis or therapeutic action. The first titer is drawn at the time of illness, the second 2 months later. The age of the patient is given in parentheses. Both tests are done at the same time.

108. _____ Rubella HAI 1:64, 1:16 (4 mo.)
109. _____ Measles HAI <1:8, 1:32 (17 yr.)
110. _____ Rubella HAI 1:16, 1:128 (29 yr., pregnant)
111. _____ Adenovirus 12 neut. <1:8, 1:64 (2 yr.)
112. _____ Anti-EBNA <1:10, 1:40 (15 yr.)
113. _____ Rubella HAI 1:16, 1:32 (29 yr., pregnant)

(a) Consider therapeutic abortion
(b) Measles
(c) Pertussis-like syndrome
(d) Infectious mononucleosis
(e) Asymptomatic reinfection, no action necessary
(f) No infection

QUESTIONS 114–120

Match the disease with its correct etiologic agent, symptom, or complication (a–g).

114. _____ Toxic shock syndrome
115. _____ AIDS
116. _____ Lyme disease
117. _____ Listeriosis
118. _____ Leprosy
119. _____ Kuru
120. _____ Onchocerciasis

(a) Facultative intracellular parasite causing meningitis
(b) Lucio's phenomenon
(c) *Staphylococcus aureus*
(d) Cerebellar ataxia
(e) *Borrelia burgdorferi*
(f) Blindness
(g) Pneumocystis pneumonia

13

The Digestive System

This is the first of a series of chapters that focus on *organ* systems of children and the things that can go wrong with them. It begins with a guide to dental problems (a much neglected area of medical education) and progresses down the alimentary tract. Many of the disorders described here have already been discussed or will be discussed later. Many diseases of children are multisystem, and thus it becomes necessary to choose one organ system chapter in which to include a disease.

Questions in this chapter may be repetitive of some from previous chapters. This is done because some of you may not be proceeding in an orderly fashion through this book, and, secondly, because some things are just worth repeating. Have fun, and don't get trapped in a blind loop.

1. Brownish discoloration of the primary teeth is seen as a result of which of the following conditions?

   (a) Hyperbilirubinemia in neonatal period
   (b) High fluoride concentration in water
   (c) Tetracycline administration
   (d) Hyperbilirubinemia and tetracycline
   (e) High fluoride and tetracycline

2. Which of the following is the principal dental problem of children in the United States?

   (a) Malocclusion
   (b) Caries
   (c) Enamel dysplasia
   (d) Delayed dentition
   (e) Supernumerary teeth

3. Factors influencing caries include each of the following EXCEPT

   (a) age
   (b) fluoride
   (c) diet
   (d) occlusion
   (e) oral hygiene

4. Each of the following is a benign condition generally requiring no treatment EXCEPT

   (a) geographic tongue
   (b) mucous retention cyst of lip
   (c) ankyloglossia
   (d) atrophic glossitis
   (e) macroglossia

5. Each of the following is suggestive of esophageal atresia EXCEPT

   (a) inability to pass a catheter into a newborn's stomach
   (b) excessive drooling of secretions
   (c) cyanosis with feedings
   (d) a gasless scaphoid abdomen
   (e) oligohydramnios

6. Which of the following statements about chalasia (gastroesophageal reflux) is true?

   (a) It has been associated with paralysis of the inferior laryngeal nerve
   (b) It is a lack of relaxation of the lower esophageal sphincter with swallowing
   (c) Surgical treatment is necessary in most infants
   (d) It often responds to putting the child in an upright position following feeding
   (e) It generally leads to iron deficiency anemia

7. Which of the following is the most common preventable cause of esophagitis in children?

   (a) Ingestion of household cleaning products
   (b) Herpes simplex virus
   (c) Diphtheria
   (d) Tuberculosis
   (e) Moniliasis

QUESTIONS 8–9

A mother calls and reports that her 15-month-old son has swallowed a coin. He tried to drink but wouldn't swallow. You tell her to bring the child to the emergency room for a roentgeno-gram. The anteroposterior projection of the chest film shows a coin facing you at the level of the aortic arch. The lateral view shows the edge of the coin.

8. The most likely place for the coin is the

(a) larynx
(b) trachea
(c) esophagus
(d) retroesophageal space
(e) anterior mediastinum

9. Treatment should be

(a) observation until the coin is vomited, coughed, or passed into the stomach
(b) direct esophagoscopy and removal of coin
(c) direct bronchoscopy and removal of coin
(d) insertion of a Foley catheter under fluoroscopy, inflation of the balloon, and removal of the coin
(e) antibiotics and steroids to prevent infection and swelling

---

10. Each of the following is true about pyloric stenosis EXCEPT

(a) The incidence is higher in males than females
(b) Onset is generally late the first month of life
(c) The vomitus is bile-stained
(d) Vomiting usually becomes projectile
(e) Jaundice occurs in association

11. The metabolic alteration found in infants with pyloric stenosis is

(a) hypochloremic acidosis
(b) hypochloremic alkalosis
(c) hyperchloremic acidosis
(d) hyperchloremic alkalosis

12. Each of the following is true of duodenal atresia EXCEPT

(a) It may be secondary to delayed vacuolization or vascular insufficiency
(b) 20 to 30% of infants with duodenal atresia have Down syndrome
(c) There is often a history of maternal polyhydramnios
(d) Classically, a "double bubble" sign is on upright film
(e) Some cases are mild, and symptoms may not be apparent until later in infancy

13. Which of the following is the most common cause of neonatal colonic obstruction?

(a) Atresia
(b) Malrotation
(c) Congenital aganglionic megacolon
(d) Meconium ileus
(e) Sigmoid stenosis

14. In distinguishing Hirschsprung disease from acquired megacolon, each of the following is useful EXCEPT

(a) size of stool
(b) symptoms present from birth
(c) palpation of feces in the abdomen
(d) presence of stool in ampulla
(e) rectal biopsy

15. Each of the following statements about Meckel diverticulum is true EXCEPT

(a) The incidence is 2 to 3%
(b) The most common presentation is abdominal pain
(c) Gastric mucosa is often present in the diverticulum
(d) Barium studies are unreliable as diagnostic tools
(e) Anemia is a common associated finding

16. Which of the following statements about duplications is NOT true?

(a) Duplications are often associated with vertebral anomalies
(b) All duplications are saccular
(c) Gastric mucosa in the duplication may lead to ulceration of adjoining normal bowel
(d) Duplications in the thorax are usually of the esophagus or stomach
(e) The most common duplication is of the ileum

17. Paralytic ileus may be caused by each of the following EXCEPT

(a) electrolyte imbalance
(b) intussusception
(c) pneumonia
(d) peritonitis
(e) appendicitis

QUESTIONS 18–20

Another late night telephone call comes from the mother of a 19-month-old infant who was fine except for an upper respiratory infection last week until 6 hours ago when he suddenly began screaming every 10 minutes. He is afebrile; he vomited twice, but had no diarrhea, although he clearly has cramping abdominal pain.

18. Which one of the following would you do?

    (a) See the child immediately
    (b) Recommend clear fluids and see the child in the morning
    (c) Prescribe an antispasmodic, anticholinergic drug and see the child if things do not improve
    (d) Suggest a tap water enema
    (e) Refer the mother to a surgeon

19. On physical examination a mass is felt in the right upper quadrant. There is bloody stool in the rectum. The most likely diagnosis is

    (a) appendicitis
    (b) gastroenteritis (shigella)
    (c) gastroenteritis (viral)
    (d) intussusception
    (e) Meckel diverticulum

20. Appropriate therapy for this disorder in most cases is

    (a) surgical resection
    (b) antibiotics and intravenous fluids
    (c) clear fluids by mouth
    (d) anticholinergic drugs
    (e) barium enema

---

21. Which of the following statements regarding high anorectal malformation in infants is true?

    (a) There is a smaller incidence of associated urinary tract anomalies as compared with low anorectal malformation
    (b) Generally there is a poorly developed anal dimple and rounded perineum
    (c) Repair is easily accomplished from below to gain continence
    (d) Females are more frequently affected than males
    (e) The internal anal sphincter is generally normal

22. Which statement is true regarding children who have had massive resection of the small intestine?

    (a) The more distal bowel preserved, the better they do

    (b) Cell-mediated immunity is impaired
    (c) The have malabsorption of water-soluble vitamins except B_{12} and folate
    (d) Clear fluids are tolerated within days of the operation

23. Each of the following is associated with a higher likelihood of peptic ulcer disease in school-aged children EXCEPT

    (a) family history of ulcer disease
    (b) being female
    (c) ingesting aspirin
    (d) high pepsinogen I levels
    (e) having type O blood

24. Which one of the following statements is true concerning peptic ulcer disease in children?

    (a) Acid secretion is increased in patients with gastric ulcers
    (b) Most gastric ulcers are found on the greater curvature
    (c) In younger children, ulcer pain is preprandial as often as it is postprandial
    (d) Antacid tablets are the most effective treatment

25. Each of the following statements is true about infections of the intestine in North America EXCEPT

    (a) "Gastroenteritis"is a misnomer
    (b) Human rotavirus accounts for most severe cases
    (c) The prevalence of bacterial infection rises in warmer climates and in areas of poor sanitation
    (d) The pathogenesis of gastroenteritis involves either invasion of the bowel wall or enterotoxin
    (e) Antibiotic treatment should begin early

26. Watery stools are characteristic in each of the following malabsorption syndromes EXCEPT

    (a) lactase deficiency
    (b) enterokinase deficiency
    (c) primary immune defects
    (d) tropical sprue
    (e) cow's milk protein sensitivity

27. Which of the following statements is true about necrotizing enterocolitis?

    (a) It is primarily a disease of infants 6 to 12 months old

(b) Breast milk feedings are protective
(c) Pneumatosis intestinalis is diagnostic
(d) Bloody stools are seen in most patients
(e) Medical management fails in 75 to 80% of cases, and surgical resection is necessary

28. Indicators of fat malabsorption include each of the following EXCEPT

(a) low serum carotene
(b) large number of fat droplets in stool
(c) high vitamin C level
(d) increased 72-hour stool fat
(e) steatorrhea

29. Each of the following tests is useful in the evaluation of malabsorption syndromes EXCEPT

(a) fecal flat balance
(b) L-xylose tolerance test
(c) stool pH
(d) hydrogen concentration in expired air
(e) blood smear

30. Which statement regarding malabsorption is true?

(a) Lactase deficiency is the most common congenital disaccharidase deficiency
(b) Watery diarrhea occurs in congenital but *not* in secondary lactase deficiency
(c) Sucrase-isomaltase deficiency may *not* lead to the presence of reducing substances in the stool
(d) Parasites cause obstruction but not malabsorption
(e) Celiac sprue is the leading cause of chronic malabsorption in children in North America

QUESTIONS 31–35

For each of the following diseases, select the specific food (a–e) that would not be absorbed well.

31. _____ Congenital lactase deficiency
32. _____ Celiac sprue
33. _____ Cow's milk protein sensitivity
34. _____ Sucrase-isomaltase deficiency
35. _____ Primary trehalase deficiency

(a) Whole wheat bread
(b) Yogurt
(c) Fruits
(d) Mushrooms
(e) Glucose water

36. Diarrhea is a presenting symptom in each of the following EXCEPT

(a) methionine malabsorption
(b) juvenile pernicious anemia (vitamin B_{12} malabsorption)
(c) acrodermatitis enteropathica
(d) primary hypomagnesemia
(e) celiac sprue

37. Which one of the following is most often confused with acute appendicitis?

(a) Crohn disease
(b) Ulcerative colitis
(c) Mesenteric adenitis
(d) Streptococcal pharyngitis
(e) Meckel diverticulum

38. Which statement is true regarding ulcerative colitis?

(a) It is most prevalent in the first decade of life
(b) Blacks are afflicted more often than whites
(c) The early lesions are transmural ulcerations of the bowel
(d) Arthritis is a common manifestation
(e) Anal fissures and ulcers are common complications

39. Each of the following has a place in the therapy of ulcerative colitis EXCEPT

(a) sulfasalazine
(b) dietary restrictions
(c) corticosteroids
(d) surgical resection

40. The most common cause of blood-stained stool in an otherwise normal infant is

(a) anal fissure
(b) anal fistula
(c) hemorrhoids
(d) Meckel diverticulum
(e) intussusception

41. Each of the following is true about inguinal hernias EXCEPT

(a) There is a higher incidence of inguinal hernias in premature infants
(b) They rarely cause pain unless incarcerated
(c) They occur only in males
(d) The treatment of choice is surgical repair
(e) The risk of incarceration and strangulation decreases with age

42. Each of the following is a cause of conjugated hyperbilirubinemia in the newborn EXCEPT

(a) Dubin-Johnson syndrome
(b) Rotor syndrome
(c) hepatitis B
(d) Crigler-Najjar syndrome
(e) benign familial cholestasis

43. Which statement about biliary atresia is true?

(a) It is potentially preventable if a hepatitis B vaccine becomes available
(b) Some cases can be corrected by the operative Kasai procedure
(c) Stools and urine are dark
(d) It is usually intrahepatic
(e) It is often associated with vitamin B_{12} deficiency

44. Persistent jaundice with hypergammaglobulinemia, a positive LE prep, anti-DNA antibodies, and an elevated transaminase are compatible with which disease?

(a) Hepatitis A
(b) Hepatitis B
(c) Chronic persistent hepatitis
(d) Chronic active hepatitis
(e) Amebic abscess

45. Each of the following may lead to cirrhosis EXCEPT

(a) Wilson disease
(b) choledochal cyst
(c) hepatitis A and B
(d) galactosemia
(e) glycogen storage disease (type I)

46. Major complications of cirrhosis include each of the following EXCEPT

(a) ascites
(b) portal hypertension
(c) encephalopathy
(d) hepatorenal syndrome
(e) hepatomegaly

QUESTIONS 47–50

At a routine 2-month check-up you note that the baby you are seeing has begun to fall off the growth curve. He was in the 50th percentile at 2 weeks of age, but the graph now indicates the 10th percentile. On questioning the mother, you find that the child has begun to vomit nearly every meal, but, although the mother (a psychiatrist) has been concerned, her gastroenterologist spouse has not. The infant is breast fed on demand and is taking no solids regularly, although the father has suggested some rice cereal to thicken the milk meal.

47. Important historical facts to be determined in this case include which of the following? (Choose as many as appropriate.)

(a) Characteristics of the vomiting (time of onset after meal, projectile, bile stained)
(b) Bowel movements
(c) Hydration (urine output, tears, etc.)
(d) Irritability or fussiness
(e) Immunization history
(f) Family medical history
(g) Social history
(h) Review of systems

48. You find that the infant has vomited forcefully nearly every feeding for the past day or so. Bowel movements are normal; urine output has been somewhat diminished. The child has been fussy. His immunizations are up to date. The father's older brother had pyloric stenosis, and the mother's brother had chalasia as an infant. The parents have been having some difficulties in their marriage and are contemplating a separation. Review of systems is noncontributory. Physical examination reveals little. A questionable mass is palpated deep in the right upper quadrant. Which one of the following would you do now?

(a) Begin a chalasia regimen and see the infant in 1 week
(b) Admit the infant for failure-to-thrive work-up
(c) Order an ultrasound of the abdomen or an upper gastrointestinal series
(d) Order an intravenous urogram
(e) Order computed tomography (CT scan) of the head

49. Gastrointestinal films reveal evidence of a "string sign." Which of the following is the most likely cause of this infant's vomiting?

(a) Chalasia
(b) Pyloric stenosis
(c) Porencephalic cyst
(d) Overfeeding
(e) Nutritional and maternal deprivation

50. Your treatment plan for this child should include which of the following? (Choose as many as appropriate.)

(a) Intravenous fluids with correction of metabolic alkalosis
(b) Upright position at all times with thickened feedings
(c) Pyloromyotomy
(d) Neurologic consultation
(e) Refer the parents to a social worker or a marriage counselor

---

51. Each of the following may have referred pain to the back EXCEPT

(a) inflammatory bowel disease
(b) duodenal ulcer
(c) pancreatitis
(d) urolithiasis
(e) appendicitis

QUESTIONS 52–60

For each of the following disorders, match the appropriate etiology or etiologic agent (a–h).

52. _____ Volvulus
53. _____ Noninflammatory cholestasis
54. _____ Microvesicular fatty liver
55. _____ Munchausen syndrome by proxy
56. _____ Byler syndrome
57. _____ Carcinoid
58. _____ Traumatic pancreatitis
59. _____ Crigler-Najjar
60. _____ Short gut syndrome

(a) Infectious
(b) Idiopathic
(c) Congenital/genetic
(d) Autoimmune/inflammatory
(e) Parent induced
(f) Drug induced/iatrogenic
(g) Tumor
(h) Iatrogenic

14

The Respiratory System

This second chapter dealing with a specific organ system concerns itself with the respiratory tract beginning with the nose and ears and ending with Ondine's curse. It repeats some of what we covered earlier in Chapters 11 and 12 but for the most part covers new material. Don't hold your breath.

1. Each of the following describes a period of morphogenesis of the fetal lung EXCEPT

(a) Embryonic
(b) Glandular
(c) Canalicular
(d) Saccular
(e) Alveolar

2. Which of the following statements is true regarding pulmonary surfactant?

(a) It is a complex mixture of glycolipids and carbohydrates
(b) It appears in the amniotic fluid approximately 1 to 2 weeks after synthesis
(c) It is synthesized by type II pneumocytes
(d) Glucocorticoids and thyroid hormone inhabit its synthesis
(e) Glucocorticoids and thyroid hormone will increase its synthesis and are of therapeutic importance

3. Which statement is true?

(a) P_{CO_2} is directly proportional to CO_2 production and alveolar ventilation
(b) Alveolar ventilation can be calculated as the difference of minute ventilation and dead space ventilation
(c) The ventilation-perfusion ratio is constant throughout the lungs
(d) The diffusion conductance for carbon dioxide is lower than that for oxygen
(e) Respiratory disease usually decreases the alveolar-arterial P_{O_2} difference

4. Each of the following is true about regulation of respiration EXCEPT

(a) The respiratory control system is a negative feedback system with a central controller

(b) The aim of respiratory regulation is to keep blood gas homeostasis in the normal range
(c) The central controller is located in the carotid bodies
(d) The efferent respiratory "organ" includes respiratory muscles
(e) Regulatory mechanisms are different in the neonate from those found in adolescents

QUESTIONS 5–10

For each of the following procedures, select the most appropriate indication (a–g).

5. _____ Bronchoscopy
6. _____ Lung biopsy
7. _____ Arterial blood gases
8. _____ Percutaneous lung tap
9. _____ Thoracentesis
10. _____ Laryngoscopy

(a) Evaluation of stridor
(b) Evaluation of pleural fluid
(c) Diagnosis of *Pneumocystis carinii* pneumonia
(d) Evaluation of atelectasis
(e) Diagnosis of infiltrate of unknown etiology not responsive to therapy
(f) Evaluation of hypercapnia
(g) Diagnosis of tuberculosis

11. Each of the following statements regarding the treatment of pediatric pulmonary disease is true EXCEPT

(a) Humidification of inspired air is an important treatment of upper airway disease
(b) Intermittent aerosols are useful for depositing medication in the lung
(c) Oxygen therapy must be accompanied by monitoring of blood gases
(d) Postural drainage is of proven value as therapy for asthma
(e) Nasotracheal tubes are more effective than cuffed endotracheal tubes in newborns

12. An arterial carbon dioxide tension ($PaCO_2$) of 45 mm Hg is least ominous in which of the following situations?

(a) cystic fibrosis
(b) epiglottitis
(c) acute asthma
(d) poisoning
(e) aspiration of a foreign body

13. Which one of the following is the most common cause of epistaxis in children?

(a) Sinusitis
(b) Polyps
(c) Thrombocytopenia
(d) Trauma
(e) Dry air

14. Each of the following statements about sinusitis in children is true EXCEPT

(a) Frontal sinusitis is most common in children under 4
(b) Symptoms may include fever, headache, and prevalent rhinitis
(c) Teeth may be tender in maxillary sinusitis
(d) Ampicillin is the antibiotic of first choice
(e) Operations are rarely necessary

15. Which of the following is true about nasal polyps?

(a) They are a common cause of epistaxis
(b) They occur commonly in patients with cystic fibrosis
(c) They are cured by steroid nasal sprays
(d) Systemic decongestants shrink most polyps
(e) Polyps are indistinguishable from swollen boggy turbinates

16. Indications for tonsillectomy include which of the following? (Choose as many as are appropriate.)

(a) Frequent sore throats
(b) Tonsils meeting in the midline
(c) Chronic airway obstruction
(d) Peritonsillar abscess
(e) Recurrent middle ear infection

17. Which of the following is true of acute nasopharyngitis in children?

(a) It is less severe than in adults
(b) The most common etiologic agent is group A strep
(c) Most children have one to two episodes a year
(d) The complications are of more clinical significance than the disease
(e) Antibiotics are useful to prevent the incidence of complications

18. Each of the following is a cause of chronic rhinitis and nasopharyngitis EXCEPT

(a) Prolonged use of topical nasal decongestants
(b) Syphilis
(c) Diphtheria
(d) Foreign body
(e) Rhinovirus

19. Which statement about laryngomalacia is true?

(a) It is usually expiratory
(b) It resolves spontaneously in most cases by the age of 1 year
(c) It is often confused with asthma in infants
(d) It is usually associated with thryoid disease
(e) It responds to oral bronchodilators

20. Each of the following is an etiologic agent for infectious croup EXCEPT

(a) measles virus
(b) parainfluenza type 2 virus
(c) *Haemophilus influenzae*, type C
(d) *Corynebacterium diphtheriae*
(e) Influenza A_2 virus

21. Each of the following is appropriate for treatment of acute viral laryngotracheobronchitis EXCEPT

(a) observation
(b) humidity
(c) antipyretics
(d) racemic epinephrine
(e) corticosteroids

QUESTIONS 22–25

A 2-year-old boy is brought to you with cough, fever, and rhinorrhea. History is unremarkable. Physical examination reveals a toxic, ill boy with fever, dyspnea, and decreased breath sounds in the left lung fields and occasional rales on the right. Posteroanterior and lateral chest films reveal an infiltrate in the left lower lobe. The right lung is clear. Leukocyte count is 19,000/cu mm with 54% PMNs, 18% band forms, and 28% lymphocytes.

22. The child is admitted to the hospital. Which of the following would you do first?

    (a) Repeat leukocyte count
    (b) Obtain a blood culture
    (c) Obtain a throat culture
    (d) Obtain a roentgenogram of the chest
    (e) Schedule bronchoscopy

23. Which antibiotic would you choose?

    (a) Methicillin
    (b) Ampicillin
    (c) Gentamicin
    (d) Penicillin G or V
    (e) Tetracycline

24. Within 24 hours he improves, and he is discharged after 3 days. He does well until 2 weeks later when 4 days after stopping antibiotics, he gets another fever, and his cough becomes worse. You should now

    (a) begin antibiotics again
    (b) order inspiratory and expiratory chest films
    (c) perform bronchoscopy
    (d) order a lung biopsy
    (e) order leukocyte count and blood culture

25. Which of the following is the most likely diagnosis?

    (a) Alpha$_1$-antitrypsin deficiency
    (b) Tuberculosis
    (c) Foreign body in the left main stem bronchus
    (d) *Pneumocystis carinii* pneumonia
    (e) Congenital lung cyst

26. Bronchiolitis in infants is most often caused by which one of the following?

    (a) Respiratory syncytial virus

    (b) Influenza virus
    (c) *Streptococcus pneumoniae*
    (d) Adenovirus
    (e) *Mycoplasma pneumoniae*

27. Which statement is true about bacterial pneumonia in children?

    (a) Bacterial infection of the lung occurs following most upper respiratory infections
    (b) Bacterial pneumonia is an unusual event in normal children
    (c) Staphylococcal pneumonia is the leading cause of pneumonia in children
    (d) Physical examination in infants is generally diagnostic, and a roentgenogram of the chest is rarely necessary
    (e) The mortality rate of pneumococcal pneumonia approaches 3 to 5%

28. Each of the following statements about staphylococcal pneumonia is true EXCEPT

    (a) It is less common than pneumococcal pneumonia
    (b) It is rapidly progressive and associated with a high morbidity and mortality
    (c) It is more common in children than in infants
    (d) Empyema, pyopneumothorax, and pneumatoceles are common
    (e) Treatment should include a semisynthetic, penicillinase-resistant penicillin and chest tube drainage if any pleural fluid is present

29. Each of the following is associated with atelectasis EXCEPT

    (a) a peanut in the bronchus
    (b) paralysis of the phrenic nerve
    (c) cystic fibrosis
    (d) asthma
    (e) Hamman-Rich syndrome

30. Pulmonary edema may be caused by each of the following EXCEPT

    (a) right ventricular failure
    (b) acute glomerulonephritis
    (c) aspiration of hydrocarbons
    (d) high altitude
    (e) hypervolemia

31. Which of the following is the most common cause of lung abscess?

    (a) Aspiration of infected material

(b) *Staphylococcus*
(c) *Nocardia*
(d) *Entamoeba histolytica*
(e) *Mycobacterium tuberculosis*

32. Pleural effusions in children are

(a) more common in males than in females
(b) most often a complication of pneumococcal pneumonia
(c) less likely to be caused by tuberculosis than they used to be
(d) usually asymptomatic
(e) easily controlled with cough suppressants

33. Which of the following is the most likely diagnosis in an otherwise normal adolescent with the sudden onset of respiratory distress, cyanosis, retractions, and markedly decreased breath sounds over the left lung?

(a) Empyema
(b) Chylothorax
(c) Left pneumothorax
(d) Staphylococcal pneumonia
(e) Aspiration of a foreign body

34. Each of the following disorders is associated with hypoventilation EXCEPT

(a) poliomyelitis
(b) myasthenia gravis
(c) pectus excavatum
(d) Guillain-Barré syndrome
(e) thoracic dystrophy

QUESTIONS 35–37

You are nearing the end of a long day in the office. It is early spring, and the winter upper respiratory season appears to have finally eased. Your last patient of the afternoon is being seen by a nurse-practitioner student you are precepting for a month. He comes out and relays the following: James, a 3-year-old, has had a cough for 2 months. It is a loose cough, but he doesn't seem to produce sputum. The cough is getting worse, especially at night. It keeps his parents awake, although James himself sleeps through the cough. Physical examination was not remarkable. Family history revealed that the mother has eczema and the father has "hay fever."

35. Additional historical facts that should be elicited to determine whether this represents a serious illness include each of the following EXCEPT

(a) reduced exercise tolerance
(b) failure to gain weight
(c) failure to grow
(d) persistent fevers
(e) recent attack of chickenpox

36. None of the additional symptoms in question 35 is present. On physical examination you hear an occasional wheeze in both lung fields. Other physical findings that would be indicative of *chronic* lung disease include which of the following? (Choose one or more.)

(a) Posterior pharyngeal drainage
(b) Hyperexpansion of the chest with an increased anteroposterior diameter
(c) Clubbing
(d) Tachypnea
(e) Cyanosis

37. James has none of the findings indicative of chronic lung disease. What would be the most likely diagnosis at this time?

(a) Bronchiectasis
(b) Pertussis
(c) Foreign body aspiration
(d) Asthma
(e) Interstitial pneumonia

QUESTIONS 38–40

Match the type of cough on the left with the etiology (a–d).

38. _____ Paroxysmal   (a) *Parainfluenza virus*
39. _____ Staccato   (b) *Bordetella pertussis*
40. _____ Croupy   (c) *Chlamydia trachomatis*
                        (d) *Mycobacterium tuberculosis*

15

The Cardiovascular System

There is nothing that commands more attention from students or residents than the heart. Hours are spent early in physical diagnosis in attempts at discerning the splitting of the first and second sounds, hearing diastolic rumbles, and identifying gallops. Whether the aura of cardiology arises out of the "life and death" nature of the heart, or the sheer numbers of cardiologists on teaching faculties (most of whom rely on technology, not stethoscopes) is not clear. Nevertheless, the field of pediatric cardiology has grown enormously in the past decade and has been linked with spectacular advances in pediatric cardiac surgery. Many children who a few decades ago would have died in infancy are now active adolescents.

This chapter will include the usual factual recall and management questions, and it will also include interpretation of electrocardiograms. Good luck, have fun, and remember the words of a wise professor who said that the stethoscope is the one instrument you could throw away and still practice pediatrics adequately.

1. The finding of substernal thrust on palpation of the precordium is most likely to be associated with which one of the following?

   (a) Left ventricular hypertrophy
   (b) Right ventricular hypertrophy
   (c) An ejection click
   (d) Systemic hypertension
   (e) Pericardial effusion

2. A Still murmur is

   (a) an early diastolic murmur signifying mitral stenosis
   (b) an innocent murmur that disappears on jugular pressure
   (c) an innocent, musical, vibratory ejection murmur heard best when the patient is in the recumbent position
   (d) an innocent, blowing, early systolic murmur that increases in intensity on expiration
   (e) a blowing diastolic murmur most frequently heard in the newborn period

3. Electrocardiograms are useful in the diagnosis of each of the following EXCEPT

   (a) congenital heart disease
   (b) rheumatic heart disease
   (c) electrolyte disorders
   (d) endocrine and metabolic disease
   (e) prematurity

QUESTIONS 4–10

The shape of the P wave is of diagnostic help in many conditions. For each of the following conditions, select the appropriate P wave shape (a–c).

4. _____ Dextrocardia
5. _____ Ebstein anomaly
6. _____ Thyrotoxicosis
7. _____ Hyperkalemia
8. _____ Tricuspid atresia
9. _____ Junctional rhythm
10. _____ Large ventricular septal defects

(a) Tall, narrow, and spiked P waves
(b) Flat P waves
(c) Inverted P waves

11. Relatively well-oxygenated blood in the fetal circulation is carried by which of the following?

    (a) Ductus venosus
    (b) Ductus arteriosus
    (c) Renal arteries
    (d) Pulmonary arteries
    (e) Umbilical arteries

12. Which statement is true?

   (a) M-mode echocardiography identifies flow
   (b) Doppler echocardiography identifies morphology
   (c) Echocardiography is useful in diagnosing prosthetic valve function
   (d) Cardiac catheterization should always follow echocardiography prior to surgery in infants with congenital heart disease
   (e) Transesophageal echocardiography has little value in the diagnosis of atrial anomalies

13. Congenital rubella syndrome is associated with which of the following?

   (a) Patent ductus arteriosus (PDA) and branch pulmonary artery stensosis
   (b) Ventricular septal defect (VSD) and PDA
   (c) Atrial septal defect (ASD) and PDA
   (d) VSD and ASD
   (e) VSD and pulmonary artery stenosis

14. Which of the following is the most common congenital heart defect in infants and children (excluding the neonatal period)?

   (a) ASD
   (b) VSD
   (c) PDA
   (d) Coarctation of the aorta
   (e) Tetralogy of Fallot

15. Tetralogy of Fallot consists of each of the following cardiac malformations EXCEPT

   (a) pulmonary stenosis
   (b) VSD
   (c) ASD
   (d) dextroposition of the aorta
   (e) right ventricular hypertrophy

16. Each of the following statements about transposition of the great arteries is true EXCEPT

   (a) It is the primary cause of death from cyanotic congenital heart disease in the first year of life
   (b) Congestive heart failure occurs by 4 months of age when a VSD is present
   (c) A VSD, PDA, and/or an ASD must be present for the newborn to survive

   (d) The electrocardiogram is often normal initially in the newborn period
   (e) More females than males are affected

17. Which of the following has improved the survival rate of infants with transposition of the great arteries?

   (a) Rashkind procedure (balloon atrial septostomy)
   (b) Echocardiography
   (c) Blalock-Taussig procedure (subclavian-pulmonary anastomosis)
   (d) Brock procedure (infundibular resection)
   (e) Home oxygen availability

18. Which one of the following is NOT present in triscuspid atresia?

   (a) Left axis deviation on electrocardiogram
   (b) Patent foramen ovale
   (c) Right ventricular hypoplasia
   (d) Split second heart sound
   (e) Diminished pulmonary vascularity on plain anteroposterior chest film

19. Which of the following statements regarding ventricular septal defect is correct?

   (a) It is most easily diagnosed at birth
   (b) Congestive heart failure usually develops within the first month of life
   (c) The defect is often small and closes spontaneously
   (d) Surgery should usually be performed within the first 6 months to prevent subacute bacterial endocarditis
   (e) Pulmonary hypertension will develop rapidly if the defect is not treated surgically

20. Which one of the following statements about atrial septal defect is true?

   (a) The murmur is caused by rapid flow from the left atrium to the right atrium
   (b) The second heart sound is variably split
   (c) High flow through the pulmonary artery causes a palpable thrill at the upper left sternal border
   (d) The defect is a patent foramen ovale
   (e) It causes heart failure in 50% of infants with the defect

21. Which of the following is the most serious atrial septal defect?

(a) Ostium primum defect
(b) Ostium secundum defect
(c) Endocardial cushion defect with common atrioventricular canal
(d) Patent foramen ovale

22. A diastolic as well as a systolic murmur in a child with a patent ductus arteriosus generally indicates which one of the following?

(a) Normal or only slightly elevated pulmonary arterial pressure
(b) Pulmonary hypertension
(c) Systemic hypotension
(d) Mitral stenosis
(e) Tricuspid stenosis

23. The majority of coarctations of the aorta occur

(a) between the origin of the right subclavian artery and the right carotid artery
(b) between the right and left carotid arteries
(c) between the left carotid artery and the left subclavian artery
(d) below the left subclavian artery
(e) at the level of the diaphragm

24. The roentgenographic finding of notching of the ribs is associated with which one of the following?

(a) Pulmonary hypertension
(b) Anomalous pulmonary venous return above the diaphragm
(c) Coarctation of the aorta

(d) Systemic hypertension
(e) Aortic insufficiency

25. In total anomalous pulmonary venous return, the anomalous vein most often enters the

(a) coronary sinus
(b) left superior vena cava
(c) right superior vena cava
(d) portal vein
(e) ductus venosus

26. The syndrome of idiopathic hypercalcemia, hypertelorism, and mental retardation is associated with which one of the following?

(a) Supravalvular aortic stenosis
(b) Valvular aortic stenosis
(c) Subvalvular aortic stenosis
(d) Aortic insufficiency
(e) Patent ductus arteriosus

QUESTIONS 27–28

A teenage girl comes to the clinic complaining that her "heart beats fast sometimes." She is otherwise well, healthy, and doing well in school. She denies taking any drugs, and she does not smoke cigarettes. Physical examination is unremarkable. Pulse rate is 80 per minute. You decide to do an electrocardiogram.

27. Below are five electrocardiograms. Which is most likely to be from this patient? (If you were to have a tracing when she is symptomatic.)

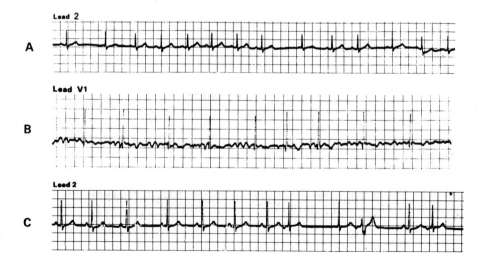

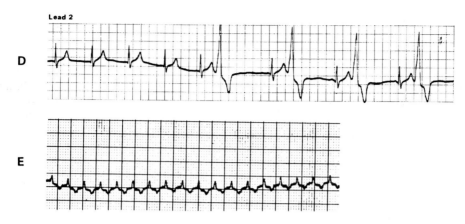

Lead 2

D

E

(From Behrman, R. E. (ed.): Nelson Textbook of Pediatrics, 14th ed. Philadelphia, W. B. Saunders Company, 1991; p. 1722; reprinted with permission.)

28. Reversion of this patient's electrocardiogram to normal will occur most readily with which of the following?

(a) Vagal stimulation
(b) Digoxin
(c) Quinidine
(d) D-C cardioversion
(e) Phenytoin (Dilantin)

29. The most common underlying factor in children who develop acute bacterial endocarditis is which of the following?

(a) Congenital heart disease
(b) Dental surgery
(c) Streptococcal pharyngitis
(d) Acute rheumatic fever
(e) Tonsillectomy

30. Which of the following is the most important procedure in the diagnosis of subacute bacterial endocarditis?

(a) Complete blood count
(b) Urinalysis (microscopic)
(c) Erythrocyte sedimentation rate
(d) Blood cultures
(e) Electrocardiogram

31. Which of the following is the most common immediate valvular lesion resulting from acute rheumatic fever?

(a) Mitral insufficiency
(b) Mitral stenosis
(c) Aortic insufficiency
(d) Aortic stenosis
(e) Tricuspid insufficiency

32. Evidence that digitalis has had an effect in an infant with congestive heart failure would include each of the following EXCEPT

(a) diminished venous pressure
(b) decreased liver size
(c) decreased P-R interval on electrocardiogram
(d) decreased heart rate
(e) increased urinary output

33. Pulsus paradoxus is associated with

(a) pericarditis
(b) endocarditis
(c) rheumatic fever
(d) myocarditis
(e) postperfusion syndrome

34. The combination of tachycardia, enlarged liver, a cardiac gallop without murmurs, and a cranial bruit is most likely

(a) congestive heart failure from viral myocarditis
(b) congestive heart failure from mucocutaneous lymph node syndrome
(c) congestive heart failure from an intracranial hemangioma
(d) thyrotoxicosis
(e) aneurysm of the circle of Willis (intracranial aneurysm)

35. Potentially curable forms of hypertension in children include each of the following EXCEPT

(a) neuroblastoma
(b) pheochromocytoma
(c) medullary cystic disease
(d) renal artery stenosis
(e) ingestion of excessive amounts of licorice

QUESTIONS 36–37

A 16-year-old girl comes to your office because of dizziness and throbbing headaches occuring two or three times a day. She has no other complaints and is otherwise in good health. There is no family history of hypertension.

36. Important other history would include which of the following? (Choose as many as are appropriate.)

(a) Renal trauma
(b) Immunizations
(c) Drug use
(d) Smoking
(e) Visual problems
(f) Nocturnal cough
(g) Personality change
(h) Excessive sweating

37. There is no history of renal trauma. Immunizations are up to date. She neither smokes nor drinks, but does take oral contraceptives. Her vision is fine, and she has no cough at all. There has been no personality change or excessive sweating. On physical examination you find that blood pressure is 140/100 mm Hg; pulse is 90 per minute; height and weight are in the 25th percentile. The remainder of the physical examination, including funduscopic examination and complete neurologic examination, is normal. There are no abdominal bruits, and her thyroid gland is normal. Which one of the following would be indicated at this point?

(a) Repeat blood pressure measurements at least twice over the next few weeks

(b) Order complete blood count, urinalysis, urine culture, and intravenous urogram
(c) Measure urinary catecholamines, 17-hydroxysteroids, and 17-ketosteroids
(d) Tell her to discontinue oral contraceptives
(e) Begin antihypertensive therapy

38. Each of the following is true about hypertension in children EXCEPT

(a) Essential hypertension is the most common form
(b) Most newborns with hypertension have hyperthyroidism
(c) Renal disease is the most likely etiology in childhood if hypertension is secondary
(d) A discrepancy in renin secretion of greater than 1.5:1 indicates renal involvement on the side with the higher level
(e) The natural history of essential hypertension is not known

39. The most common cardiac tumor in childhood is

(a) rhabdomyosarcoma
(b) mesothelioma
(c) papilloma
(d) lipoma
(e) myxoma

QUESTIONS 40–45

For each of the drugs listed below, select the mechanism of action (a–e).

40. _____ Phentolamine
41. _____ Verapamil
42. _____ Minoxidil
43. _____ Propranolol
44. _____ Clonidine
45. _____ Hydralizine

(a) Arteriolar dilatation
(b) B-receptor blockade
(c) Calcium channel blocker
(d) 2-α agonist in CNS
(e) α-receptor blockade

16
Diseases of the Blood

This chapter reviews the hematologic system. It covers anemia, blood cell disorders, coagulopathies, and platelet and white cell functions. It is an important subject, since anemias of various types are very common in pediatric practice. In addition, a wealth of new knowledge in the area of coagulation defects has accumulated very rapidly, and now nearly 1 in 20 of us has some form of von Willebrand disease.

The questions in this chapter are of varying types, including the usual clinical management problem. Nowhere will we ask whether blood is thicker than water.

1. The predominant hemoglobin present a birth in normal infants is

   (a) hemoglobin A
   (b) hemoglobin A_2
   (c) hemoglobin F
   (d) hemoglobin Gower
   (e) hemoglobin Portland

2. Each of the following functions of the ATP generated by red cells from glucose metabolism is necessary for RBC viability EXCEPT

   (a) Maintenance of electrolyte gradients
   (b) Initiation of energy production
   (c) Maintenance of red cell membrane size and shape
   (d) Maintenance of heme iron in the ferric form
   (e) Maintenance of the levels of organic phosphates

3. The hematocrit is normally at its lowest level at which age in childhood?

   (a) 1 hour
   (b) 1 week
   (c) 1 month
   (d) 3 months
   (e) 3 years

4. Each of the following is true about congenital pure red cell anemia (Diamond-Blackfan syndrome) EXCEPT

   (a) Levels of hemoglobin F are increased for age
   (b) Erythropoietin activity is high
   (c) Corticosteroid therapy is beneficial if begun early
   (d) Hemosiderosis is a common sequela
   (e) Spontaneous remission occasionally occurs

5. Which one of the following statements about megaloblastic anemia is true?

   (a) A goat's milk diet may often cause it
   (b) The peak incidence is at 2 years of age
   (c) Rickets often accompanies the disease
   (d) When present at 4 to 7 months, vitamin B_{12} deficiency is the usual cause
   (e) The reticulocyte level is usually high

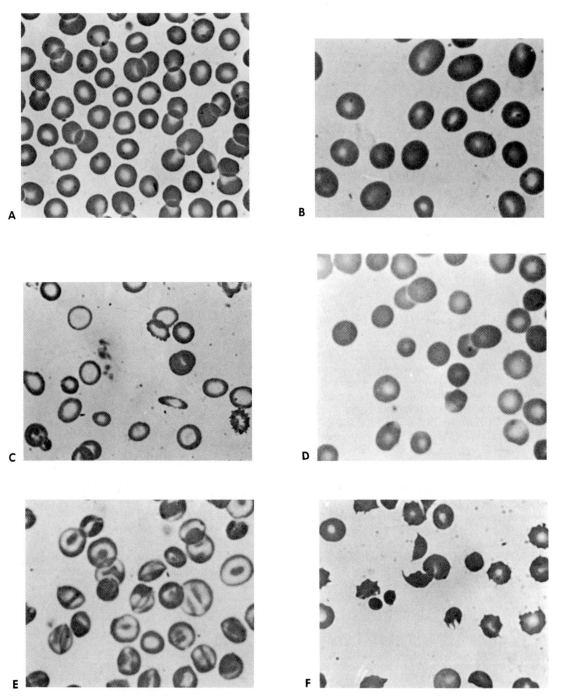

(From Behrman, R. E. (ed.): Nelson Textbook of Pediatrics, 14th ed. Philadelphia, W. B. Saunders Company, 1991; p. 1237, reprinted with permission.)

6. Blood smear *B* above demonstrates macrocytes. Each of the following is compatible with the smear shown EXCEPT

(a) celiac disease
(b) chronic blood loss
(c) pregnancy
(d) juvenile pernicious anemia
(e) methotrexate treatment for leukemia

7. A heat-lable protein in cow's milk has been associated with which one of the following?

(a) Transient erythroblastoma of child-
    hood
(b) Transcobalamine II deficiency
(c) Iron deficiency anemia
(d) Folic acid deficiency
(e) Juvenile pernicious anemia

QUESTIONS 8–10

For these questions, choose as many lettered
choices as applicable. *All, some, or none may
be correct.*

8. Which of the following hemolytic anemias
   is/are caused by enzymatic defects of the
   red cells?

   (a) Pyruvate kinase deficiency
   (b) Drug-induced hemolytic anemia
   (c) Hexokinase deficiency
   (d) Sickle cell anemia

9. Characteristics of glucose-6-phosphate dehydrogenase (G-6-PD) deficiency include
   which of the following?

   (a) High incidence in American black males,
       Italians, and Greeks
   (b) Autosomal dominant inheritance pat-
       tern
   (c) Sulfonamides, naphthaquinolones, and
       antipyretics may precipitate hemolysis
   (d) Affected persons have 50% or less of
       G-6-PD activity

10. Which of the following statements about
    sickle cell anemia is/are true?

    (a) Vaso-occlusive episodes are the most
        frequent type of sickle cell crisis
    (b) Sequestration crises occur primarily in
        adults
    (c) Patients are highly susceptible to pneu-
        mococcal diseases
    (d) The diagnosis is made conclusively by
        a rapid slide test

11. Pallor, hemosiderosis, jaundice, and extra-
    medullary hematopoiesis are characteristics
    of which one of the following disorders?

    (a) Sickle cell trait
    (b) Sickle cell anemia
    (c) Thalassemia minor
    (d) Thalessemia major
    (e) Hemoglobin C-thalassemia

12. Polycythemia in childhood may result from
    each of the following EXCEPT

    (a) living at high altitude
    (b) right-to-left shunts
    (c) dehydration following severe burns
    (d) congenital methemoglobinemia
    (e) Down syndrome in newborns

13. Each of the following has been used in the
    treatment of children with constitutional
    aplastic anemia (Fanconi syndrome) EX-
    CEPT

    (a) estrogens
    (b) transfusion
    (c) antibiotics
    (d) androgens
    (e) corticosteroids

QUESTIONS 14–20

Mark "T" if the statement is true, "F" if it is
false.

14. _____ The major indications for blood
    transfusion are to treat shock follow-
    ing acute blood loss and to provide
    red blood cells for maintenance of
    blood hemoglobin level
15. _____ Transfusion is indicated for a child
    with chronic iron deficiency anemia
    and a hemoglobin of 8 gm/dl
16. _____ Platelet transfusion is often given
    without regard to ABO or Rh type
17. _____ With the advent of testing for hep-
    atitis B antigen, hepatitis has disap-
    peared as a complication of blood
    transfusion
18. _____ Urticaria occurs in 1 to 2% of pa-
    tients receiving transfusion
19. _____ Congestive heart failure precipitated
    by transfusion is more likely in a pa-
    tient with chronic anemia than in a
    patient with acute hemorrhage
20. _____ Normal blood, if fresh (1 to 2 days
    old), is an adequate source of white
    blood cells.

21. The absolute number of neutrophils con-
    sidered to be normal in infants and young
    children is

    (a) 100 to 1500/cu mm
    (b) 1500 to 2500/cu mm

(c) 2500 to 6000/cu mm
(d) 6000 to 12,000/cu mm
(e) >12,000/cu mm

22. Neutropenia is characteristic of each of the following EXCEPT

(a) stress
(b) Bodian-Schwachman syndrome
(c) rubella
(d) influenza B
(e) typhoid fever

23. In chronic granulomatous disease, the neutrophils are

(a) markedly decreased in number
(b) unable to increase their numbers in response to a bacterial infection
(c) incapable of intracellular killing of certain bacteria
(d) leukemoid in number
(e) able to reduce nitroblue tetrazolium (NBT) dye

24. Each of the following blood factors is involved in the intrinsic coagulation system EXCEPT

(a) factor VII
(b) factor VIII
(c) factor IX
(d) factor XI
(e) factor XII

25. Each of the following statements is true about factor VIII deficiency EXCEPT

(a) Clinical severity is inversely proportional to the plasma level of factor VIII
(b) In severe cases hemarthrosis and large intramuscular hematomas are common
(c) The partial thromboplastin time is prolonged
(d) Administration of fresh citrate phosphate dextrose (CPD)-preserved blood stops hemorrhage
(e) Aspirin is contraindicated

26. An infant is scheduled for an elective herniorrhaphy. Routine coagulation screen prior to the operation reveals a normal platelet count and partial thromboplastin time, but a markedly prolonged prothrombin time. Deficiency of which of the following factors is most likely?

(a) II, V, VIII, X
(b) II, V, VII, X

(c) V, VII, VIII, X
(d) VIII, IX, XI, XII
(e) IX, X, XI, XII

QUESTIONS 27–30

For each disease, select the associated factor deficiency (a–e).

27. _____ Hemophilia A   (a) Factor VI
28. _____ Hemophilia B   (b) Factor VIII
29. _____ Hemophilia C   (c) Factor IX
30. _____ Hageman factor   (d) Factor XI
              deficiency   (e) Factor XII

---

31. Each of the following is true about hemorrhagic disease of the newborn EXCEPT

(a) It is usually self-limited, with only a small percentage of infants being severely affected
(b) Breast milk contains enough vitamin K to prevent it
(c) Manifestations such as melena, umbilical stump bleeding, or hematuria usually begin 48 to 72 hours after birth
(d) Vitamin K given at birth will prevent it
(e) It rarely occurs after the neonatal period

QUESTIONS 32–35

32. An 18-month-old Caucasian boy is brought to your office for a routine health maintenance visit. Things are going well according to the mother; she has no concerns. You notice that the child is in the 60th percentile for height and weight and the 50th percentile for head circumference. Further questioning of the mother reveals that the child always appears hungry; in fact, he drinks a quart of whole milk a day and also eats dirt and other objects. Intake of solid foods is sporadic, but the mother states that she thought all 18-month-olds were "picky eaters." Physical examination reveals mild pallor of the conjunctivae. There is no hepatosplenomegaly, and the rest of the examination is normal. Based on the information, which of the following would be the most likely to determine the diagnosis?

(a) Complete blood count, including blood smear
(b) Reticulocyte count

(c) Lead screen

(d) Ophthalmologic consultation

(e) Testing stools for occult blood

33. The smear shows a microcytic, hypo-chromic anemia. Iron supplementation therapy is started. When will the reticulocyte response be maximum?

(a) 1 to 2 days

(b) 5 to 7 days

(c) 14 to 21 days

(d) 3 to 4 weeks

(e) About 6 weeks

34. When the hemoglobin and hematocrit return to normal, which should be done?

(a) Stop iron supplementation

(b) Continue iron for 1 to 2 weeks

(c) Continue iron for 4 to 8 weeks

(d) Continue iron for 4 to 6 months

35. If the boy's anemia does not improve, which of the following should be explored? (Choose as many as are appropriate.)

(a) Gastrointestinal blood loss

(b) Thalassemia

(c) Sickle cell anemia

(d) Urinary tract infection

(e) Parasitic infection

36. Each of the following statements concerning the spleen is true EXCEPT

(a) It is palpable in 5 to 10% of normal children

(b) Splenomegaly from venous obstruction (Banti syndrome) is most commonly associated with liver disease

(c) It has vascular, lymphatic, and lymphoreticular components

(d) Congenital asplenia as an isolated anomaly is known as the Ivemark syndrome

(e) Functional hyposplenia most commonly occurs in children with sickle cell disease

37. Which of the following statements regarding children who have had splenectomy is/are true? (Choose as many as are appropriate.)

(a) *Haemophilus influenzae* infection is the leading bacterial complication

(b) The incidence of overwhelming sepsis is highest in children who have had splenectomy for hereditary spherocytosis

(c) Howell-Jolly bodies are seen in the blood smear

(d) Immunization with polysaccharide antigens reduces the risk of pneumococcal sepsis

(e) Older children are at greater risk of sepsis than are infants

QUESTIONS 38–45

For each of the following disorders, select the appropriate platelet presentation (a–c).

38. _____ Anaphylactoid purpura

39. _____ Aspirin toxicity

40. _____ ITP

41. _____ Wiskott-Aldrich syndrome

42. _____ Kawasaki disease

43. _____ DIC

44. _____ TTP

45. _____ Kasabach-Merritt syndrome

(a) Platelets decreased in number

(b) Platelet count normal

(c) Platelets increased

QUESTIONS 46–50

For each of the conditions below, match the battery of laboratory values given (a–e).

46. _____ DIC

47. _____ Liver disease

48. _____ Vitamin K deficiency

49. _____ Classic von Willebrand disease

50. _____ Type IIB von Willebrand disease

(a) Prolonged bleeding time, increased restocetin-induced platelet aggregation (RIPA)

(b) Prolonged PPT, PT, TT, and Factor VII

(c) Prolonged PTT, PT, Normal TT, Factor VII

(d) Prolonged bleeding time, reduced RIPA

(e) Prolonged PTT, PT, TT, decreased Factor VIII

17

Neoplasms and Neoplasm-Like Lesions

If you spend much time in tertiary care or university hospitals as a student or resident, you would think that neoplastic diseases in children were as common as pneumonia. Cancer is the leading cause of death by disease in children, and many inpatient facilities have two to three children at a time receiving treatment for neoplastic disease. It has been gratifying to watch the marked reduction in mortality rates, especially in childhood leukemia, but as long as the etiologies of cancer remain obscure, prevention will be a dream, not a reality.

This chapter covers the neoplastic diseases of children. The format does not include the usual management questions, since most of us should refer, not treat, neoplasia in children.

1. Which one of the following statements is true?

(a) Cancer is the leading cause of death in children
(b) Environmental factors play a role in 60 to 90% of childhood neoplasms
(c) Leukemia is the most common cancer in children
(d) Ewing sarcoma is more prevalent in black than in white children
(e) Burkitt lymphoma is common in black children in the United States

QUESTIONS 2-10

For each of the following tumor types or syndrome, match the chromosome associated with it (a-f).

2. _____ Retinoblastoma   (a) 5q
3. _____ Wilms tumor   (b) 10q
4. _____ Hepatoblastoma and   (c) 11p
        Beckwith-Wiedemann   (d) 13q
5. _____ Multiple endocrine neo- (e) 17q
        plasia type 2A   (f) 22q
6. _____ Neurofibromatosis-1
7. _____ Neurofibromatosis-2
8. _____ Familial polyposis and
        colorectal cancer
9. _____ Osteosarcoma
10. _____ Rhabdomyosarcoma

QUESTIONS 11-16

For each drug, select the major mode of action (a-f).

11. _____ Methotrexate   (a) Inhibits purine
12. _____ Epipodophyl-   biosynthesis
        lotoxins   (b) Inhibits DNA-
13. _____ 6-Mercapto-   dependent
        purine   RNA synthesis
14. _____ Bleomycin   (c) DNA strand
15. _____ Actinomycin   scission
        D   (d) Inhibits tetra-
16. _____ Asparaginase   hydrofolate
                                      synthesis
                                 (e) Premitotic cell/
                                      cycle delay
                                 (f) Inhibits pro-
                                      tein synthesis

QUESTIONS 17-20

For each drug, select the potentially irreversible, dose-related toxicity (a-d).

17. _____ Asparaginase   (a) Leukoenceph-
18. _____ Bleomycin   alopathy
19. _____ Methotrexate   (b) Myocardial
20. _____ Anthracy-   damage
        clines   (c) Pancreatitis
                                 (d) Pulmonary
                                      fibrosis

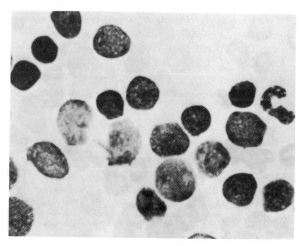

(From Behrman, R. E. (ed.): Nelson Textbook of Pediatrics, 14th ed. Philadelphia, W. B. Saunders Company, 1991; p. 1300; reprinted with permission.)

21. The bone marrow above shows

(a) infectious mononucleosis
(b) effect of treatment with asparaginase
(c) chronic myelocytic leukemia
(d) acute lymphocytic leukemia
(e) acute nonlymphocytic leukemia

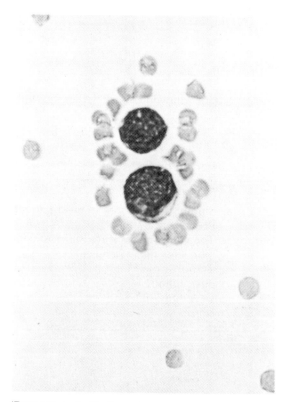

(From Mauer, A. M.: Current treatment of acute leukemia. Compr. Ther., *4*:58, 1979; reprinted with permission.)

22. This finding, shown at bottom left, with sheep erythrocytes is characteristic of

(a) chronic lymphocytic leukemia
(b) T-cell form of ALL
(c) B-cell from ALL
(d) "null"-cell form of ALL
(e) acute myelocytic leukemia

23. Which of the following forms of acute lymphocytic leukemia has the best prognosis?

(a) B cell
(b) T cell
(c) Pre-B cell
(d) "Null"-cell form
(e) All are about the same

24. Hodgkin disease occurs primarily in

(a) newborns
(b) infants
(c) preschool-aged children (2 to 5 years old)
(d) school-aged children (5 to 12 years old)
(e) adolescents

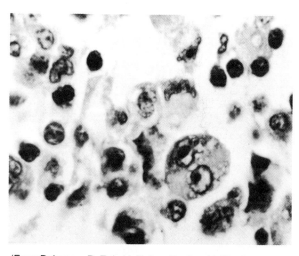

(From Behrman, R. E. (ed.): Nelson Textbook of Pediatrics, 12th ed. Philadelphia, W. B. Saunders Company, 1991; p. 1301; reprinted with permission.)

25. The large cell with two nuclei in the lower right quadrant of this section of lymph node biopsy above is diagnostic of

(a) B-cell form of acute lymphocytic leukemia
(b) chronic myelocytic leukemia
(c) Hodgkin disease
(d) neuroblastoma
(e) histiocytosis

26. Each of the following statements about neuroblastoma is true EXCEPT

    (a) Most of these tumors arise in the abdomen
    (b) Metastatic disease is common at the time of diagnosis
    (c) Thoracic tumors are generally found in the posterior mediastinum
    (d) The younger the infant at the time of diagnosis, the worse the prognosis
    (e) Urinary vanillylmandelic acid is usually increased

27. A high incidence of genitourinary anomalies has been associated with which of the following tumors?

    (a) Wilms tumor
    (b) Neuroblastoma
    (c) Pheochromocytoma
    (d) Osteosarcoma
    (e) All of the above

28. Which of the following is the most common soft tissue sarcoma in children?

    (a) Fibrosarcoma
    (b) Hemangiosarcoma
    (c) Rhabdomyosarcoma
    (d) Synovial sarcoma
    (e) Liposarcoma

29. Each of the following statements is true of BOTH osteosarcoma and Ewing sarcoma EXCEPT

    (a) The tumor occurs in the second decade of life
    (b) The most frequent presenting symptom is pain
    (c) Metastases occur in the lung
    (d) Amputation of the affected extremity is the treatment of choice
    (e) Chemotherapy is an adjunctive therapy

30. A rare tumor occurring predominantly in black children associated with Epstein-Barr virus is

    (a) hepatocarcinoma
    (b) retinoblastoma
    (c) adenocarcinoma of the rectum
    (d) nasopharyngeal carcinoma
    (e) adenocarcinoma of the vagina

31. Which one of the following benign tumors does NOT usually require surgery or curettage?

    (a) Osteoid osteoma
    (b) Osteoblastoma
    (c) Nonossifying fibroma
    (d) Enchondroma

32. Leukokoria is the initial presentation of which of the following?

    (a) Chondrosarcoma
    (b) Retinoblastoma
    (c) Nasopharyngeal carcinoma
    (d) Optic glioma
    (e) Chronic lymphocytic leukemia

33. An intraembryonic tissue tumor with all three germ cell types is the

    (a) seminoma
    (b) embryonal cell carcinoma
    (c) teratocarcinoma
    (d) choriocarcinoma
    (e) Sertoli tumor

QUESTIONS 34–40

For each o the following, mark "A" if the statement is true about hemangiomas only, "B" if it is true about lymphangiomas only, "C" if it is true of both, or "D" if true of neither.

34. _____ Benign tumor
35. _____ Congestive heart failure is a complication
36. _____ Surgery is necessary in most patients
37. _____ Prednisone suppresses tumor growth
38. _____ The head and neck are the most common sites of occurrence
39. _____ Tumor growth may result in airway obstruction
40. _____ Peak tumor growth occurs in adolescence

18

The Urinary System and Pediatric Gynecology

We review here Chapter 18 of the textbook, The Urinary System and Pediatric Gynecology. It begins with the anatomy of the glomerulus and covers the important area of renal physiology before progressing through the urinary tract. The section on pediatric gynecology is quite brief, 0.4% of the textbook. The topic is more important than that and the brevity of the section may reflect the discomfort many pediatric professionals seem to have in examining the area.

Both patient management questions and the usual multiple choice questions will be found here. Have fun, and don't get caught in the loop of Henle.

QUESTIONS 1–4

Choose the *one* best answer.

1. Each of the following is a part of the nephron EXCEPT

    (a) glomerulus
    (b) juxtaglomerular apparatus
    (c) proximal convoluted tubule
    (d) loop of Henle
    (e) collecting duct

2. The formula

$$\frac{(\text{urinary concentration of solute}) (\text{urinary flow rate})}{\text{plasma concentration of solute}} \times$$

    measures

    (a) renal clearance
    (b) renal plasma flow
    (c) renal blood flow
    (d) tubular secretion
    (e) tubular reabsorption

3. Each of the following may color the urine red EXCEPT

    (a) blackberries
    (b) urates
    (c) homogentisic acid
    (d) myoglobin
    (e) beets

4. Each of the following is a glomerular cause of hematuria EXCEPT

    (a) Alport syndrome
    (b) membranous glomerulopathy
    (c) Goodpasture disease
    (d) hypercalciuria
    (e) anaphylactoid purpure

5. The predominant pathogenetic mechanism for glomerular injury is

    (a) genetic (biochemical)
    (b) immunologic
    (c) coagulopathy
    (d) traumatic
    (e) infectious

6. The predominant immunoglobulin deposited in the glomeruli of patients with Berger nephropathy is

    (a) IgA
    (b) IgD
    (c) IgE
    (d) IgG
    (e) IgM

7. Which statement is true about acute glomerulonephritis following streptococcal pharyngitis?

    (a) It is most common in the summer months
    (b) Its incidence is the same in boys and girls

(c) Pharyngeal infection with a nephrito-
genic strain of streptococci leads to acute
glomerulonephritis more than 50% of
the time
(d) Early treatment of the pharyngitis reduces the likelihood of acute glomerulonephritis
(e) Second attacks of glomerulonephritis are
common

8. Complications of acute poststreptococcal
glomerulonephritis include each of the following EXCEPT

(a) hyperkalemia
(b) hypernatremia
(c) encephalopathy
(d) pulmonary edema
(e) anuria

9. Depressed serum complement (C3) levels
are found in each of the following EXCEPT

(a) acute poststreptococcal glomerulonephritis
(b) proliferative glomerulonephritis secondary to septicemia
(c) membranous lupus nephritis
(d) focal proliferative lupus nephritis
(e) the nephritis of anaphylactoid purpura

10. The triad of microangiopathic hemolytic
anemia, renal failure, and thrombocytopenia is characteristic of which one of the
following?

(a) Membranous lupus nephritis
(b) Focal glomerulonephritis secondary to
septicemia
(c) Hemolytic uremic syndrome
(d) Acute poststreptococcal glomerulonephritis
(e) Berger disease

QUESTIONS 11–13

For each of the following, *one* or *more than one*
answer may be correct.

11. Which is/are present in the nephrotic syndrome?

(a) Edema
(b) Hypoproteinemia
(c) Increased tubular reabsorption of sodium
(d) Decreased serum cholesterol and triglycerides

12. The minimal lesion form of the nephrotic
syndrome (lipoid nephrosis) is diagnosed
by the finding(s) of

(a) systemic hypertension
(b) retraction of epithelial foot processes
on glomerular basement membrane
(c) hypocomplementemia
(d) selective proteinuria

13. Tubular pathologic causes of proteinuria include

(a) fever
(b) exercise
(c) vitamin D intoxication
(d) sarcoidosis
(e) heavy metal poisoning

QUESTIONS 14–15

Choose the *one* best answer.

14. Which one of the following is the first-line
treatment for the minimal lesion form of
the nephrotic syndrome in children?

(a) Prednisone
(b) Chlorambucil
(c) Cyclophosphamide
(d) Prednisone and chlorambucil
(e) Prednisone and cyclophosphamide

15. Which of the following pairs of M streptococcal serotypes is MOST commonly associated with acute poststreptococcal glomerulonephritis?

(a) 1, 2
(b) 4, 6
(c) 12, 49
(d) 25, 52
(e) 49, 57

QUESTIONS 16–24

For each of the following, mark "D" if the
characteristic is associated with *d*istal type of
renal tubular acidosis, "P" if it is associated
with *p*roximal renal tubular acidosis, or "B" if
it is associated with *b*oth types, or "M" if associated with *m*ineralocorticoid deficiency.

16. _____ Hereditary
17. _____ Addison disease

18. _____ Amphrotericin B
19. _____ Lead poisoning
20. _____ Toluene sniffing
21. _____ Hyperparathyroidism
22. _____ Sickle cell nephropathy
23. _____ Galactosemia
24. _____ Outdated tetracycline

QUESTIONS 25–40

Choose as many answers as appropriate. *One or more* may be correct.

25. Which of the following statements about nephrogenic diabetes insipidus is/are true?

    (a) It is an X-linked recessive disorder
    (b) Administration of vasopressin results in increased urinary osmolality in patients with this disorder
    (c) Initial manifestations include fever, constipation, and failure to thrive
    (d) A high-protein, low-salt diet is the most important therapeutic regimen
    (e) Hydrochlorothiazide is useful in its treatment

26. Polyuria and polydipsia are symptoms of which of the following disorders?

    (a) Diabetes mellitus
    (b) Renal glycosuria
    (c) Nephrogenic diabetes insipidus
    (d) Hypercalcemia
    (e) Distal renal tubular acidosis

27. Which of the following statements about Bartter syndrome is/are true?

    (a) The etiology is unknown, but is related to a primary defect in chloride reabsorption in the loop of Henle
    (b) Hypokalemia is a constant feature
    (c) Prognosis is uniformly poor and all patients develop renal failure
    (d) Older children, present with growth retardation
    (e) Licorice and diuretic misuse need to be differentiated in diagnosis

28. Cystic changes of clinical significance are found in *both* the liver and kidney in which of the following disorders?

    (a) Oxalosis
    (b) Nephronophthisis

    (c) Nail-patella syndrome
    (d) Childhood-type (autosomal recessive) polycystic kidney disease
    (e) Adult-type (autosomal dominant) polycystic kidney disease

29. Prerenal causes of acute renal failure in children (out of the newborn period) include which of the following?

    (a) Hemolytic uremic syndrome
    (b) Congenital renal obstruction (e.g., unrethral valves)
    (c) Acute leukemia
    (d) Shock
    (e) Acute poststreptococcal glomerulonephritis

30. Which of the following is/are usually present in acute renal failure?

    (a) Hypokalemia
    (b) Hyponatremia
    (c) Hypocalcemia
    (d) Hypophosphatemia
    (e) Metabolic acidosis

31. Hemodialysis is preferred to peritoneal dialysis in which of the following circumstances?

    (a) Blood urea nitrogen greater than 125 mg/dl
    (b) Uncontrollable hyperkalemia
    (c) Intractable lactic acidosis
    (d) Barbiturate intoxication
    (e) Methanol intoxication

32. Which of the following statements about chronic renal failure (CRF) in children is/are true?

    (a) The essential feature of CRF is a decreased glomerular filtration rate
    (b) Clinical problems do not usually appear until 70% of renal function is lost
    (c) In infants, CRF is usually caused by glomerular disease
    (d) The principal renal anomalies causing CRF are renal hypoplasia and bilateral vesicoureteral reflux
    (e) The incidence of CRF in infants is about the same in females and males

33. Which of the following is/are found in patients with chronic renal failure?

    (a) Hypoglycemia following an oral glucose load

(b) Prolonged bleeding time
(c) Secondary hyperparathyroidism
(d) Normochromic anemia
(e) Hypersecretion of gastric acid

34. Which of the following drugs require(s) modified dosage in children with renal failure?

(a) Penicillin
(b) Gentamicin
(c) Digoxin
(d) Acetaminophen
(e) Thiazides

35. Which of the following statements concerning acute pyelonephritis is/are true?

(a) Frequency, urgency, and dysuria are presenting symptoms in older children
(b) High fever, chills, and flank pain generally occur in children
(c) Red blood cell casts appear in the urine
(d) In the newborn period the infection is usually hematogenous in origin
(e) Significant vesicoureteral reflux is a common associated finding

36. Which of the following statements about cryptorchidism is/are true?

(a) Approximately 17% of low birth weight infants (2000 to 2500 g) are cryptorchid
(b) Spontaneous descent is unusual after 1 year of age
(c) Intravenous urogram and voiding cystourethogram should be performed because of an increased incidence of urinary anomalies
(d) In bilateral cryptorchidism, urinary gonadotropins are lower than normal
(e) Elective orchidopexy should be performed during the third year of life

37. Which of the following statements about urinary lithiasis is/are true?

(a) The condition is more common outside the United States
(b) Calcium carbonate stones predominate
(c) Struvite stones follow urinary tract infections
(d) Lithotriptor treatment alone is all that is necessary
(e) Surgical removal is rarely necessary

38. Vulvovaginitis in a 5-year-old may be caused by

(a) *Gardnerella vaginalis*
(b) *Candida albicans*
(c) *Enterobius vermicularis*
(d) bubble bath
(e) herpes genitalis

39. Prepubertal vaginal bleeding is associated with which of the following?

(a) Traumatic injury
(b) Prolapse of the urethral mucosa
(c) Streptococcal vaginitis
(d) Precocious puberty
(e) Sarcoma botryoides

40. Which of the following statements about adenocarcinoma of the vagina in young women is/are true?

(a) There is an association with the mother's use of diethylstilbestrol during her pregnancy
(b) Vaginal bleeding is a frequent presenting sign
(c) The Pap smear is diagnostic and as reliable as it is for carcinoma of the cervix
(d) Adenovirus and herpesvirus are etiologic
(e) Surgical treatment is indicated

QUESTIONS 41–44

41. An infant is admitted to the hospital because of vomiting and lethargy. The child shows evidence of failure to thrive, and physical examination reveals an abdominal mass. Blood and urinary cultures grow *Escherichia coli*. The most likely cause of this disorder is

(a) mesenteric cyst
(b) Wilms tumor
(c) adrenal hemorrhage
(d) obstruction at the ureteropelvic junction
(e) retrocaval ureter

42. An adolescent boy notices a painless "ropelike" mass in the left side of the scrotum. The most likely diagnosis is

(a) epididymitis
(b) torsion of an appendage
(c) torsion of the testis
(d) hydrocele
(e) varicocele

43. A breast mass in an adolescent female is least likely to be

(a) fibroadenoma
(b) adenocarcinoma
(c) abscess
(d) fat necrosis
(e) fibrocystic disease

44. A mother and her 15½-year-old caucasian daughter come to you because the young woman has not begun to menstruate. Medical history and complete physical examination are normal. Breast development and pubic hair have been present for 18 months and are normal. Which would be most appropriate?

(a) Reassurance that she likely will begin menstruating within the year
(b) Laboratory evaluation for systemic disease
(c) Urinary estriol determination
(d) Buccal smear
(e) Referral for psychologic counseling

QUESTIONS 45–50

The telephone rings at 5:30 PM as you are about to leave for the weekend. It is Mr. Johnson, a single parent of a 3-year-old girl, who tells you that the child is complaining of burning on urination and she is urinating frequently. He stresses the importance of clearing this up quickly since he has a busy weekend ahead.

45. Which of the following questions is/are pertinent at this point? (Choose as many as are appropriate.)

(a) Does she have fever?
(b) Has she used bubble bath recently?
(c) Has she been scratching her anus, or waking up at night restless and crying?
(d) Does she have blurred vision or headaches?
(e) Is there blood in her urine?

46. Based on the answers he gives you, as well as his clear distress, you suggest that he bring her to the office. Physical examination is remarkable only for mild costovertebral angle tenderness, mild suprapubic tenderness, and some periurethral-erythema. Temperature is 37.5° C (99.5° F). Appro-

priate evaluation would include which of the following? (Choose as many as are appropriate.)

(a) Complete blood count
(b) Urinalysis
(c) Urinary culture
(d) Throat culture
(e) Intravenous urogram
(f) Voiding cystourethrogram

47. Results of laboratory studies (whether or not indicated in 51):

Hematocrit	41%
Hemoglobin	13.5 gram/dl
Leukocyte count	8800/cu mm; 40% segmented neutrophils; 3% band forms; 56% lymphocytes; 1% monocytes
Urinalysis	Cloudy urine; pH 6.0; protein and acetone trace, glucose negative; 50–100 WBCs, 10–15 RBCs/hpf; numerous bacteria; no casts

Throat and urinary cultures are started. Other studies are scheduled.

Based on the information obtained so far, the most likely diagnosis is

(a) nonspecific urethritis
(b) lower urinary tract infection
(c) acute pyelonephritis
(d) chronic pyelonephritis
(e) benign familial hematuria

48. The most appropriate treatment would be

(a) sitz baths and forced fluids
(b) trimethoprim-sulfamethoxazole orally twice a day
(c) ampicillin, parenterally
(d) nitrofuratoin macroscrystals (Macrodantin), orally 2 times daily
(e) reassurance only

49. Follow-up should include which one of the following?

(a) Repeat urinalysis and urinary culture Monday and in 14 to 21 days
(b) Intravenous urogram and voiding cystourethrogram when infection subsides
(c) Chronic use of nitrofurantoin

(d) Careful monitoring of blood pressure and urinary output

(e) No follow-up is necessary

50. Several weeks after cessation of antibiotics she has another UTI. After treatment, an IVP is done (right). The diagnosis and appropriate treatment are

(a) grade I reflux; antibiotic Rx only prophylactically

(b) grade II reflux; symptomatic Rx

(c) reflux and paraureteral diverticulum; symptomatic Rx

(d) reflux and paraureteral diverticulum; surgical Rx

(e) normal; no Rx

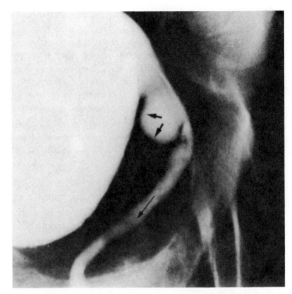

(From Behrman, R. E. (ed.): Nelson Textbook of Pediatrics, 14th ed. Philadelphia, W. B. Saunders Company, 1991; p. 1365; reprinted with permission.)

19
The Endocrine System

This chapter in the Review will cover the endocrine system and will include disorders of the pituitary, thyroid, parathyroid, and adrenal glands, as well as the gonads.

Biochemistry, physiology, and genetics all interface in these pages, and an understanding of all of them will make endocrinology less confusing. Nevertheless, the interrelationships of the various hormonal systems are complex and not easy to understand on first reading. This review should help you sort things out. We will continue with multiple choice questions and a management problem or two to keep the rest in perspective. Try not to get depressed if you cannot remember all the intricacies of steroid chemistry and gonadal hormonal function and dysfunction.

1. Which of the following statements regarding the endocrine system is/are true? (More than one may be correct.)

   (a) Somatostatin is a hypothalamic hormone that inhibits the secretion of somatotropin
   (b) All hypothalamic secretions are either releasing hormones or inhibitory hormones
   (c) Pituitary hormones act on other endocrine glands but do *not* affect individual cells in the rest of the body
   (d) Pituitary thyrotropin production is inhibited by a hypothalamic hormone
   (e) The function of the posterior pituitary is controlled by neurosecretions rather than directly by hypothalamic secretions

2. A 10-year-old child stops growing and has signs of hypothyroidism. The most likely *nonthyroid* etiology for this condition is

   (a) craniopharyngioma
   (b) hypothalamic tumor
   (c) tuberculosis
   (d) sarcoidosis
   (e) aneurysm of the circle of Willis

3. Which *one* of the following statements about growth hormone (GH) is true?

   (a) Levels rise at about 4 PM and fall after sleep
   (b) Exercise stimulates GH release
   (c) Administration of L-dopa inhibits GH release

   (d) Low serum levels of GH rule out primary hypothyroidism
   (e) Administration of hGH will reduce levels of somatomedin-C

QUESTIONS 4–5

A child is below the third percentile for height. Growth velocity is normal, but chronologic age is greater than skeletal age.

4. This condition is called

   (a) primary hypopituitarism
   (b) secondary hypopituitarism
   (c) constitutional delay in growth
   (d) genetic short stature
   (e) primordial dwarfism

5. The growth hormone levels in this child are most likely

   (a) elevated
   (b) normal
   (c) depressed
   (d) variable

6. Short stature, voracious appetite, and insomnia in a child are characteristic of which one of the following?

   (a) Laron syndrome
   (b) Primary hyperthyroidism
   (c) Diabetes mellitus
   (d) Deprivation dwarfism
   (e) Diabetes insipidus

7. Silver syndrome includes which of the following? (Choose one or more.)

   (a) Congenital asymmetry
   (b) Short stature
   (c) Small genitalia
   (d) Decreased excretion of gonadotropins
   (e) Accelerated bone maturation

8. Each of the following statements about diabetes insipidus (arginine vasopressin deficiency) is true EXCEPT

   (a) Polyuria and polydipsia are the main symptoms
   (b) Destruction of the supraoptic and paraventricular nuclei leads to diabetes insipidus
   (c) It is hereditary in a minority of cases
   (d) The disease can be differentiated from nephrogenic diabetes insipidus by measuring the response to exogenous vasopressin
   (e) Amelioration of symptoms usually indicates that the disease has been cured

9. Which of the following is the most effective treatment of inappropriate secretion of antidiuretic hormone?

   (a) Infusion of hypertonic saline (3%)
   (b) Restriction of fluids
   (c) Chlorpropamide, orally
   (d) Demeclocycline, orally
   (e) Mannitol by intravenous infusion

10. Which of the following statements about true precocious puberty is/are correct? (Choose one or more.)

   (a) It is always isosexual
   (b) The cause is never found in most cases
   (c) Patients are taller than average adults
   (d) Unless associated with a tumor, it is usually harmless
   (e) Medroxyprogesterone acetate (Provera) is the treatment of choice

11. Which of the following statements concerning hypothyroidism is/are true?

   (a) The presence of maternal thyroxine prevents hypothyroidism in the fetus
   (b) Maternal ingestion of propylthiouracil often leads to neonatal goiter
   (c) Developmental defects of the thyroid gland are the most common causes of congenital hypothyroidism
   (d) Children with deiodinase deficiency excrete enough iodine in their urine to cause hypothyroidism
   (e) Thyrotropin deficiency is the most common cause of acquired hypothyroidism

12. Which of the following statements regarding congenital hypothyroidism is/are true?

   (a) Girls and boys are affected with equal frequency
   (b) Breast feeding protects infants from severe hypothyroidism
   (c) Retardation of bone growth and development does not appear until 3 to 4 months of age
   (d) Prolonged "physiologic" jaundice is a clue to the diagnosis
   (e) Wormian bones are often seen on roentgenograms of the skull

13. Which of the following statements regarding goiter is/are true?

   (a) It usually results from elevated thyrotropic hormone
   (b) It does not occur in euthyroid children
   (c) It most often occurs in the United States as a result of iodine-deficient diet
   (d) Ectopic thyroid tissue is susceptible to goitrous enlargement
   (e) It is almost always present in congenitally hyperthyroid infants

14. Lymphocytic thyroiditis can be differentiated from simple goiter by which of the following? (Choose one or more.)

   (a) Clinical observation
   (b) Determination of antithyroid antibody-titer (immunofluorescent technique)
   (c) Measurement of serum thyroid stimulating hormone
   (d) Measurement of serum thyroxine
   (e) Therapeutic trial with thyroid extract

15. A 10-year-old child is noted to have lagging of the upper eyelid when she looks down. Her eyes cannot converge, and there is retraction of her upper eyelid. This constellation of signs is diagnostic of (choose one)

   (a) lymphocytic thyroiditis
   (b) congenital hypothyroidism
   (c) simple goiter
   (d) Graves disease
   (e) solitary thyroid nodule

16. Characteristics of congenital hyperthyroidism include which of the following? (Choose one or more.)

    (a) Higher prevalence in girls than in boys
    (b) History of Graves disease in the mother
    (c) Cranial synostosis
    (d) Resolution of symptoms by 3 months of age
    (e) Cardiac failure (high-output) in severe cases

17. Immediate surgery for a solitary thyroid nodule is indicated in which of the following situations? (Choose one or more.)

    (a) A thyroid mass that has been present for 2 years suddenly enlarges
    (b) The nodule is "cold" on technitium scan
    (c) The nodule is hard
    (d) The vocal cords are involved
    (e) Adjacent lymph nodes are enlarged

18. The substance of choice for maintenance therapy of hypoparathyroidism is oral administration of (choose one)

    (a) parathyroid hormone extract
    (b) calcium supplements
    (c) vitamin D_2
    (d) magnesium sulfate
    (e) CaEDTA

19. Each of the following is associated with parathyroid adenoma EXCEPT (choose one)

    (a) muscular weakness
    (b) normal parathyroid hormone levels
    (c) nephrocalcinosis
    (d) hypercalcemia
    (e) polydipsia and polyuria

20. The most common etiology of Addison disease in children is

    (a) tuberculosis
    (b) histoplasmosis
    (c) amyloidosis
    (d) metastatic carcinoma
    (e) autoimmune destruction

QUESTIONS 21–22

An infant is brought to the emergency room with vomiting, lethargy, dehydration, and failure to thrive. Intravenous administration of fluids is begun. Serum electrolyes are sodium 124 mEq/l, chloride 88 mEq/l, and potassium 6.8 mEq/l. Serum glucose is 35 mg/dl. The child is hypotensive and has areas of depigmentation.

21. The most likely diagnosis is

    (a) Addison disease
    (b) Waterhouse-Friderichsen syndrome
    (c) 17-hydroxylase deficiency
    (d) Cushing syndrome
    (e) adrenoleukodystrophy

22. Treatment for this infant should include which of the following? (Choose as many as are appropriate.)

    (a) Desoxycorticosterone acetate (DOCA)
    (b) Hydrocortisone hemisuccinate
    (c) Adrenalectomy
    (d) Insulin
    (e) Glucagon

23. The most common form of congenital adrenal hyperplasia is deficiency of

    (a) 3-β-hydroxysteroid dehydrogenase
    (b) 11-β-hydroxylase
    (c) 17-hydroxylase
    (d) 21-β-hydroxylase
    (e) aldosterone

24. Which of the following is/are associated with adrenocortical tumors? (Choose one or more.)

    (a) Masculinization of girls
    (b) Pseudoprecocious puberty in boys
    (c) Hemihypertrophy
    (d) Normal levels of urinary 17-ketosteroids
    (e) Genitourinary anomalies

25. Each of the following is true about pheochromocytoma in children EXCEPT

    (a) The tumor arises from the chromaffin cells
    (b) Tumors are usually right-sided
    (c) When coexisting with neurofibromatosis it is known as Sipple syndrome
    (d) Hypertension is a common symptom
    (e) Urinary VMA is increased

26. Gynecomastia is common in all of the following EXCEPT

    (a) newborns
    (b) young children

(c) pubescent children
(d) patients with Klinefelter syndrome
(e) patients receiving digitalis

27. Stein-Leventhal syndrome is characterized by each of the following EXCEPT

(a) amenorrhea
(b) hirsutism
(c) infertility
(d) hypertension
(e) obesity

28. Each of the following is associated with gonadal defects EXCEPT

(a) 47, XXX genotype
(b) deletion of the short arm of the Y chromosome
(c) XY pure gonadal dysgenesis

(d) deficiency of steroid 5-α-reductase
(e) true hermaphroditism

29. Swyer syndrome is an example of

(a) Male pseudohermaphroditism
(b) Female pseudohermaphroditism
(c) True hermaphroditism
(d) Testicular feminization

30. Features which differentiate Noonan syndrome from Turner syndrome include which of the following? (More than one answer may be correct.)

(a) Pulmonary valvular defect instead of aortic
(b) Normal chromosomal configuration
(c) Occurs in males only
(d) Associated with mental retardation
(e) Sexual maturation occurs

20

Neurologic and Muscular Disorders

As the end of the Textbook nears, chapters become shorter. Rather than have minichapters of 10 to 15 questions in the Review, we will merge two or more Textbook chapters into one Review chapter. In keeping with that plan, this part of the Review will cover The Nervous System and Neuromuscular Diseases.

Whether it is because of the incredible complexity of the nervous system, or the fact that evolution has left us unique among the species in cortical development, these subjects always seem awesome. Neurology itself seems to be at a stage where description outweighs therapeutics—so many disorders can only be palliated, and many others only described. We are often left in the position of doing our best to diagnose and support those who come to us with neuromuscular problems rather than being able to treat the problem definitively or know that it will go away.

The format remains the same, but the degree of difficulty will be inversely proportional to the prevalence of the disorder. Don't worry if you don't do as well here as before.

1. Which of the following statements concerning convulsions in children is/are true? (Choose one or more.)

   (a) Infection is the most common cause of convulsions in the neonatal period
   (b) Febrile convulsions usually occur between 6 and 60 months of age
   (c) Idiopathic epilepsy first appears as an important cause of convulsions in the third year of life
   (d) During midchildhood, congenital brain defects are the primary causes of convulsions
   (e) Infection is the most common cause of convulsions in adolescence

2. Which of the following statements regarding neonatal seizures is/are true? (Choose one or more.)

   (a) Grand mal seizures commonly follow birth anoxia
   (b) Maternal drug use during pregnancy can cause seizures in the newborn
   (c) The prognosis is generally poor for newborns with seizures
   (d) The symptoms are variable, and the electroencephalogram may be the only way of detecting seizures
   (e) Treatment includes general supportive measures and phenobarbital or diazepam

3. A child has a febrile seizure. Which of the following would be associated with a *poor* prognosis? (Choose one or more.)

   (a) The seizure lasted more than 1 hour
   (b) The patient has shigellosis
   (c) Five more seizures occur within a year
   (d) The electroencephalogram remains abnormal for 48 hours following the seizure
   (e) The patient is 17 months old and has been receiving phenobarbital since he had a febrile seizure 8 months ago

4. A mother describes her 5-year-old daughter as being "intelligent," but says she has occasional "lapses" during which she will "not be here" and "drop things." What is the most likely diagnosis?

   (a) Grand mal seizures
   (b) Petit mal seizures
   (c) Focal seizures
   (d) Myoclonic seizures
   (e) Psychomotor seizures

5. *Abnormal* electroencephalographic patterns in children include which of the following? (Choose one or more.)

(a) Multiple, high-voltage spikes over the right parietal area
(b) 1 to 2 per second, high-voltage spike and wave patterns
(c) 3 to 8 per second slow rhythms
(d) 14 to 16 per second positive spikes
(e) 8 to 12 per second alpha waves

6. Which of the following is/are true about status epilepticus? (Choose one or more.)

(a) The most common cause is head trauma in an epileptic child
(b) Intravenously administered diazepam is effective treatment
(c) Phenobarbital, 1 to 2 mg/kg intramuscularly, is effective treatment
(d) Failure to control status within 60 minutes should institute a prompt search for another organic lesion
(e) Inhalation anesthesia can be used as an adjunct to treatment in most cases

7. In the long-term management of seizure disorders in children, which of the following is/are correct?

(a) An adolescent patient should not participate in sports
(b) Children and parents should be told that medication must be continued for at least 3 to 4 years
(c) The child should be encouraged to participate in regular activities
(d) The family should be reassured that the epileptic child is normal and will probably grow out of the disorder

8. Which of the following is/are correct regarding sodium valproate? (Choose one or more.)

(a) It is replacing phenobarbital and phenytoin as a first-line treatment for grand mal seizures
(b) It has sedative side effects
(c) It probably inhibits gamma aminobutyric acid transaminase
(d) It is very effective against psychomotor seizures

QUESTIONS 9–16

For each therapeutic measure listed on the left, select the seizure disorder(s) (a–d) that it is effective against. (One or more might apply.)

9. _____ Phenobarbital   (a) Grand mal

10. _____ Phenytoin   (b) Petit mal
        (Dilantin)   (c) Psychomotor
11. _____ Carbamazepine   (d) Infantile
        (Tegretol)   myoclonic
12. _____ Primidone
        (Mysoline)
13. _____ Ethosuximide
        (Zarontin)
14. _____ Trimethadione
        (Tridione)
15. _____ Ketogenic diet
16. _____ ACTH

17. Which of the following statements regarding the prognosis in seizure disorders is/are true? (Choose one or more.)
(a) Convulsions rarely cause cerebral damage
(b) Acute grand mal seizures become more numerous unless treated
(c) Spontaneous remission of grand mal epilepsy occurs
(d) Children with petit mal tend to have higher intelligence quotients than those with other types of seizures
(e) Children with epilepsy are better adjusted if their parents also have epilepsy

18. Which of the following is/are increased in patients with upper motor neuron lesions? (Choose one or more.)

(a) Strength
(b) Muscle tone
(c) Coordination
(d) Tendon reflexes
(e) Involuntary movements

19. Involuntary movements are associated with lesions in which of the following locations? (Choose one or more.)

(a) Upper motor neurons
(b) Basal ganglia
(c) Cerebellum
(d) Anterior horn cells
(e) Peripheral nerves

20. A lesion in which one of the following sites will lead to bitemporal hemianopsia?

(a) Right optic nerve
(b) Right optic tract
(c) Left visual cortex
(d) Left lateral geniculate body
(e) Optic chiasm

21. Which of the following reflexes is/are normally present in a 5-month-old infant? (Choose one or more.)

(a) Moro reflex
(b) Placing reflex
(c) Stepping reflex
(d) Tonic neck reflex
(e) Plantar grasp reflex

QUESTIONS 22–28

For each disorder listed on the left, select the most likely neurologic findings (a–d) for a patient in coma.

22. _____ Arteriovenous malformation
23. _____ Lead poisoning
24. _____ Drug intoxication
25. _____ Reye syndrome
26. _____ Brain tumor (left parietal)
27. _____ Subdural hemorrhage (in an infant)
28. _____ Hydrocephalus

(a) No focal signs, normal intracranial pressure (ICP)
(b) No focal signs, increased ICP
(c) Focal signs, normal ICP
(d) Focal signs, increased ICP

29. Which of the following statements about spina bifida occulta is/are true? (Choose one or more.)

(a) It is most common at L3 and L4
(b) It can be seen as an incidental finding in about 20% of roentgenograms of the spine
(c) The most common defects are unilateral foot deformity and weakness of the foot muscles
(d) The impairments worsen over time
(e) Dermoid cysts are present in about half the cases

30. Causes of communicating hydrocephalus include which of the following? (Choose one or more.)

(a) Arnold-Chiari malformation
(b) Aqueductal stenosis
(c) Dandy-Walker malformation
(d) Papilloma of choroid plexus
(e) Midline brain tumor

31. The leading cause of cerebral palsy in the United States is

(a) kernicterus
(b) cerebral infection at birth
(c) cerebral anoxia at birth
(d) hydrocephaly
(e) epilepsy

32. Which is/are true about migraine headaches?

(a) An aura precedes the headache in the classic case
(b) The pain is bilateral in most cases
(c) Laboratory studies are helpful in the differential diagnosis
(d) Vasoconstrictors usually prevent an attack if given at the onset of symptoms
(e) Attacks rarely recur if phenobarbital is used as long-term maintenance therapy

33. A child with a seizure disorder has brownish-red nodules in a "butterfly" distribution over the face. The most likely diagnosis is

(a) neurofibromatosis
(b) Sturge-Weber disease
(c) tuberous sclerosis
(d) systemic lupus erythematosus
(e) von Hippel-Lindau disease

34. Degenerative diseases of cerebral gray matter include (choose one or more)

(a) Tay-Sachs disease
(b) Friedreich ataxia
(c) multiple sclerosis
(d) Krabbe disease
(e) Niemann-Pick disease

35. Cerebellar ataxia, spastic weakness, optic neuritis, and diplopia are common presenting symptoms of which one of the following?

(a) Schilder disease
(b) Neuromyelitis optica
(c) Metachromatic leukodystrophy
(d) Multiple sclerosis
(e) Muscular dystrophy

36. Which one of the following ataxic disorders is associated with a specific immunologic dysfunction?

(a) Friedreich ataxia
(b) Ataxia-telangiectasia

(c) Roussy-Lévy syndrome
(d) Abetalipoproteinemia
(e) Refsum syndrome

QUESTIONS 37–38

In the late fall, you are asked to see a 7-year-old boy who has a 3-week history of progressively worsening headaches. They are most severe in the morning. He has vomited intermittently over the last 2 days, but denies nausea. He has done poorly in school this year, and lately he has refused to go because of the headaches. There has been no fever, diarrhea, upper respiratory infection, or any other symptoms. Physical examination is unremarkable except for slight blurring of the optic discs and mild hypotonia of the right arm and leg.

37. The most likely diagnosis is

   (a) brain tumor
   (b) pseudotumor cerebri
   (c) school phobia
   (d) lead encephalopathy
   (e) Reye syndrome

38. If this were a brain tumor, what would it most likely be?

   (a) Cerebellar astrocytoma
   (b) Ependymoma
   (c) Pontine glioma
   (d) Craniopharyngioma
   (e) Optic glioma

---

39. Which of the following is/are true about Reye syndrome? (Choose one or more.)

   (a) It is associated with influenza B infection
   (b) Its symptoms are similar to those of severe salicylism
   (c) Children who survive usually recover within 2 to 3 days
   (d) Anticonvulsants and phenothiazines are indicated for treatment
   (e) The incidence has declined

40. Which of the following statements concerning closed head trauma in children is/are true? (Choose one or more.)

   (a) A blow causing dizziness and nausea is likely to be serious even if it did not cause unconsciousness

(b) Retrograde amnesia is often seen in children with concussion
(c) The presence of skull fracture always implies significant underlying brain injury
(d) Epidural hemorrhage usually results from severance of the middle meningeal artery
(e) Chronic subdural hematomas in infants most often result from abuse or birth trauma

41. Which of the following is/are found in familial dysautonomia (Riley-Day syndrome)? (Choose one or more.)

   (a) Elevated urinary vanillylmandelic acid
   (b) Decreased urinary homovanillic acid
   (c) Positive Mecholyl test (pupil)
   (d) Negative (no wheal) histamine skin test
   (e) Diminished pressor response to norepinephrine

42. Anterior horn cell diseases include (choose one or more)

   (a) infantile spinal muscular atrophy (Werdnig-Hoffman disease)
   (b) poliomyelitis
   (c) Guillain-Barré syndrome
   (d) familial dysautonomia (Riley-Day syndrome)
   (e) atonic diplegia

43. Proximal progression of paralysis that is symmetrical is characteristic of which of the following? (Choose one or more.)

   (a) Poliomyelitis
   (b) Acute coxsackievirus infection
   (c) Guillain-Barré syndrome
   (d) Charcot-Marie-Tooth disease
   (e) Hypertrophic interstitial neuritis

44. A child has vesicular and papular lesions on the right side of the face, pain and hyperacusis of the right ear, and loss of taste on the anterior two thirds of the tongue. The most likely diagnosis is

   (a) Tolosa-Hunt syndrome
   (b) Bell palsy
   (c) sixth nerve palsy
   (d) Erb-Duchenne paralysis
   (e) otitis media and cellulitis

45. A previously health 10-year-old girl develops double vision, which worsens as the day progresses. Examination reveals ptosis which increases while she gazes upward. Which of these statements is/are true about her condition? (Choose one or more.)

    (a) Her mother probably also has this condition
    (b) The symptoms will probably be transient
    (c) The problem may be the result of food poisoning
    (d) It is surprising for this condition to occur in a girl
    (e) Anticholinesterase drugs are indicated

46. An infant is brought to you because he looks only to the right, and the mother has noted a mass in the right side of the neck. Which of the following statements about this condition is/are true? (Choose one or more.)

    (a) If not treated, asymmetry of the face is likely to develop
    (b) The mass is probably a rhabdomyosarcoma
    (c) Treatment consists of simple stretching exercises only

    (d) The erythrocyte sedimentation rate, serum creatine phosphokinase level, and leukocyte count are probably elevated
    (e) The condition was probably caused by trauma

47. A 4-year-old child has difficulty in climbing stairs, slow motor development, and hypertrophied calf muscles. The most likely diagnosis is

    (a) myasthenia gravis
    (b) myotonia congenita
    (c) Duchenne muscular dystrophy
    (d) hypokalemic periodic paralysis
    (e) central core disease

QUESTIONS 48–50

For each of the conditions listed, match the therapeutic agent of choice (a–d), if any.

48. _____ Tolosa-Hunt syndrome
49. _____ Familial periodic paralysis
50. _____ Myotonia congenita

    (a) Acetazolamide
    (b) Procainamide
    (c) Corticosteroids
    (d) No treatment available

21

Disorders of the Eye and Ear

This is a short but difficult chapter with a lot of material, some very important to pediatricians, some not. Attentive longtime readers of the Textbook and Review will notice that, in this edition, the ear was appended to the eye. Visualize that metaphor! Instead of management problems, questions about funduscopic pictures are included. These are meant to stimulate you to look at children's fundi. The only way to become familiar with what the fundus looks like is to look at the fundus. That may sound obvious, but I know many students and residents who don't examine newborn or infant fundi "because they are too hard to see." Along with the tympanic membranes of newborns, the fundi may be the last examined of all body parts. Both are examinable, however, and for those of you who don't try, the prophecy of "never seeing it" will be self-fulfilling.

1. Which of the following statements about the term newborn eye is/are true? (Choose one or more.)

   (a) A bluish tinge to the sclera is indicative of osteogenesis imperfecta
   (b) The lens is flatter than in older children
   (c) The fundus is less pigmented than in later life
   (d) Retinal hemorrhages are present in up to 25% of newborns
   (e) Fixation and visual acuity are present beginning at 2 to 4 weeks of age

2. The majority of newborns have physiologic (choose one)

   (a) hyperopia
   (b) myopia
   (c) emmetropia
   (d) astigmatism
   (e) anisometropia

3. Which of the following statements about myopia in childhood is/are true? (Choose one or more.)

   (a) The image falls posterior to the retina
   (b) The far point of clear vision varies directly with the degree of myopia
   (c) Frowning and squinting are common manifestations

   (d) Concave lenses will correct the problem
   (e) The condition has a hereditary tendency

4. Causes of amblyopia include (choose one or more)

   (a) macular scarring secondary to trauma in one eye
   (b) uncorrected anisometropia
   (c) strabismus
   (d) myopia
   (e) hyperopia

5. Emergency ophthalmologic evaluation is indicated in which of the following situations? (Choose one or more.)

   (a) Nyctalopia in a school-aged child
   (b) Amaurosis (present since birth) in an infant
   (c) Amaurosis in a previously well child
   (d) Sudden onset of diplopia in an adolescent
   (e) Dyslexia in a school-aged child

6. A preverbal child suddenly begins to tilt his head to the right and to close one eye while reading. Which statement(s) about this case is/are correct?

   (a) There is probably paralysis of the right superior oblique muscle

(b) Diplopia probably exists
(c) The child probably has accommodative esotropia
(d) An operative procedure will be curative
(e) Treatment should include patching one eye

7. In a child with left esotropia, which of the following is/are true? (Choose one or more.)

   (a) The Hirschberg test will be positive
   (b) The esotropia may be secondary to epicanthal folds
   (c) Covering the right eye will cause the left eye to move outward
   (d) Covering the left eye will cause the right eye to move outward
   (e) Uncovering the left eye will cause the right eye to move inward

8. Surgical intervention is indicated in which of the following? (Choose one or more.)

   (a) Congenital ptosis
   (b) Epicanthal folds
   (c) Entropion
   (d) Hordeolum
   (e) Coloboma

9. Common conditions of newborns include which of the following? (Choose one or more.)

   (a) Chalazion
   (b) Dacryocystitis
   (c) Dacryoadenitis
   (d) Alacrima
   (e) Opsoclonus

10. Which of the following is the most common etiologic agent for ophthalmia neonatorum?

    (a) *Neisseria gonorrhoeae*
    (b) *Chlamydia oculogenitalis*
    (c) *Hemophilus* species
    (d) *Streptococcus pneumoniae*
    (e) *Staphylococcus aureus*

11. The fundus shown top right is most compatible with which of the following?

    (a) Glaucoma
    (b) Toxoplasmosis

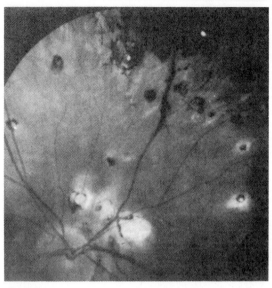

(From Behrman, R. E. (ed.): Nelson Textbook of Pediatrics, 14th ed. Philadelphia, W. B. Saunders Company, 1991; p. 1587).

(c) Retrolental fibroplasia
(d) Retinitis pigmentosa
(e) Dislocation of the lens

12. Retrolental fibroplasia is most likely the result of

    (a) local retinal anoxia secondary to hyperoxemic vasoconstriction
    (b) oxygen toxicity to the rods and cones
    (c) retinal detachment
    (d) vasoproliferation secondary to hypoxemia
    (e) sympathetic ophthalmia

13. Which of the following statements about the condition shown on p. 108 (top) is/are true? (Choose one or more.)

    (a) It is usually bilateral
    (b) It results from cytomegalovirus infection
    (c) The most common presenting sign is a white "cat's eye" reflex in the pupil
    (d) It is highly malignant
    (e) It usually occurs in adolescents

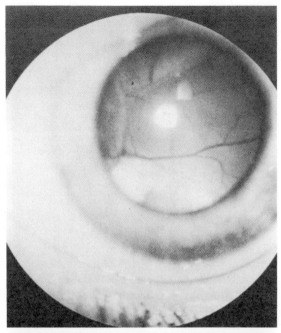

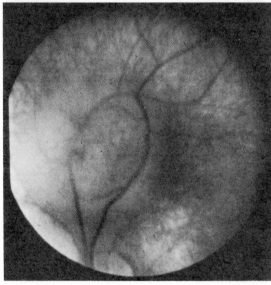

(From Behrman, R. E. (ed.): Nelson Textbook of Pediatrics, 14th ed. Philadelphia, W. B. Saunders Company, 1991; p. 1590; reprinted with permission.)

14. The fundus on p. 109 (top left) is most likely from a child with

(a) congenital infection
(b) trauma to the eye
(c) neurodegenerative disease
(d) hypertension
(e) tuberous sclerosis

15. Which of the following statements regarding orbital cellulitis is/are true? (Choose one or more.)

(a) Infection occurs by venous extension
(b) Anaerobes are the most common pathogens
(c) Cavernous sinus thrombophlebitis may be a sequela
(d) Topical antibiotics are mandatory
(e) Occasionally, surgical drainage is required

16. A 6-month-old child with the fundus depicted on p. 109 (bottom left) should be (choose one)

(a) treated with antimicrobials
(b) given antihypertensive therapy
(c) reported to appropriate welfare authorities
(d) given a reduced inspired oxygen level
(e) operated on for a tumor

17. Which of the following ophthalmic solutions is most likely to be effective in the treatment of herpes keratitis?

(a) 5-iodo-2-deoxyuridine
(b) Hydrocortisone
(c) Zephrian chloride
(d) 10% Sodium sulfacetamide
(e) Cyclopentolate hydrochloride

QUESTIONS 18–25

Match the disease or syndrome on the left with the ophthalmologic manifestation on the right (a–f).

18. ____ Morquio syndrome	(a)	Congenital glaucoma
19. ____ Tay-Sachs disease	(b)	Corneal clouding
20. ____ Tuberous sclerosis	(c)	Hypertelorism
21. ____ Wilson disease	(d)	Macular cherry red spot
22. ____ Pierre Robin syndrome		
23. ____ Niemann-Pick disease	(e)	Retinal phakomata
24. ____ Seckel syndrome	(f)	Kayser-Fleischer ring
25. ____ Congenital rubella		

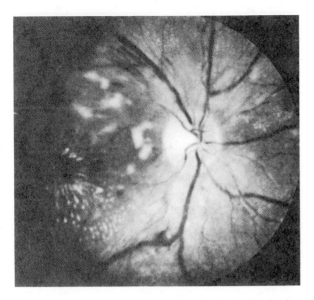

(From Behrman, R. E. (ed.): Nelson Textbook of Pediatrics, 14th ed. Philadelphia, W. B. Saunders Company, 1991; p. 1592; reprinted with permission.)

26. Which of the following statements is/are true with regard to hearing loss in children and infants?

    (a) Hearing loss will affect 3% of children by age 6

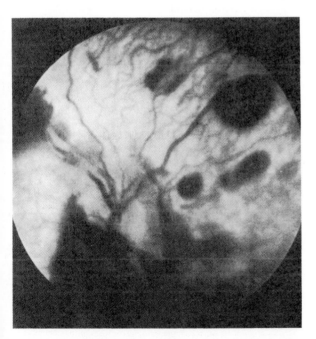

(From Behrman, R. E. (ed.): Nelson Textbook of Pediatrics, 14th ed. Philadelphia, W. B. Saunders Company, 1991; p. 1599; reprinted with permission.)

    (b) Hearing loss in infants and children is usually central in origin

    (c) Approximately 50% of cases of moderate to severe hearing loss are genetically determined

    (d) Most familial hearing impairment of the sensineural type is X-linked

27. Newborn hearing screening is indicated for each of the following EXCEPT

    (a) Neonatal asphyxia
    (b) Neonatal meningitis
    (c) Hyperbilirubinemia requiring exchange transfusion
    (d) Neonatal otitis media
    (e) Congenital rebella or CMV infection

QUESTIONS 28–30

For each question below, answer "A" if the answer matches Figure A, "B" if Figure B or "C" if neither.

28. _____ Serous otitis media
29. _____ Sensineural hearing loss
30. _____ Normal findings

A

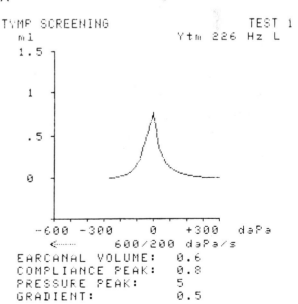

(From Behrman, R. E. (ed.): Nelson Textbook of Pediatrics, 14th ed. Philadelphia, W. B. Saunders Company, 1991; p. 1606.)

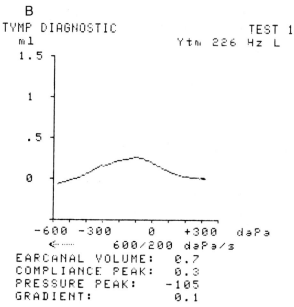

B

TYMP DIAGNOSTIC   TEST 1
ml   Ytm 226 Hz L

1.5

1

.5

0

    -600 -300   0   +300   daPa
    <------   600/200 daPa/s
EARCANAL VOLUME: 0.7
COMPLIANCE PEAK: 0.3
PRESSURE PEAK: -105
GRADIENT: 0.1

(From Behrman, R. E. (ed.): Nelson Textbook of Pediatrics, 14th ed. Philadelphia, W. B. Saunders Company, 1991; p. 1607.)

31. Each of the following is true about the auditory brain stem response (ABR) EXCEPT

    (a) It is useful for neonatal hearing screening
    (b) It is affected adversely by general anesthesia
    (c) In older children it is *not* a "hearing test"
    (d) Sedation has no effect on results
    (e) It is recorded as five to seven waves

32. Which statement is true?

    (a) The inner ear reaches adult size in the middle of fetal development
    (b) The middle ear arises from the 3–4 branchial arch
    (c) Anotia is a common minor deformity
    (d) Pit depressions should be surgically removed

    (e) Congenital malformations of the inner ear are common and associated with sensorineural hearing loss

33. Each of the following organisms is an etiologic agent for otitis externa. Which one is most common?

    (a) *Staphylococcus epidermides*
    (b) *Streptococcus pyogenes*
    (c) *Proteus*
    (d) *Pseudomonas*
    (e) *Candida albicans*

QUESTIONS 34–39

Match the symptom or physical finding on the left with the most likely organism on the right (a–f).

34. _____ Furunculosis   (a) *Pseudomonas*
35. _____ Acute cellulitis   (b) *Staphylococcus aureus*
36. _____ Otitis media (chronic supporative)   (c) Strep pneumoniae
37. _____ Ramsay-Hunt syndrome   (d) Strep pyogenes
38. _____ Bullous myringitis   (d) Herpes simplex
39. _____ Otitis media (acute)   (f) Herpes zoster

40. Perforation of the tympanic membrane by trauma (choose the best answer)

    (a) Should be treated with antibiotics topically
    (b) Are more likely to heal if caused by compression injury than a penetrating injury
    (c) Usually requires tympanoplastic surgery
    (d) Usually occurs in the inferior portion of the pars tensa when caused by compression

22
Bones, Joints, and Skin

For many years the education of pediatric residents in dermatology and orthopedics was sorely lacking in many training programs. Practicing pediatricians know that these two areas are extremely important in the "real world," so careful attention should be paid to Chapters 23 and 24 of the textbook. In spite of some orthopedists' protests that all problems of bones and joints should be referred to them, it is still the pediatrician or family physician who is usually consulted first. (We charge less, too!) So, until such time as parents rush directly to orthopedic surgeons, we should make an effort to learn as much as we can about orthopedics. This is true for dermatology as well.

We will rely a little more on pictures in this chapter for obvious reasons. Note that since the last edition the order of chapters in the Textbook has been reversed, with dermatology moving ahead of orthopedics. If you wish to follow that order slavishly, begin with questions 30–65, then do 1–29. Questions 1 and 2 relate to the following figure:

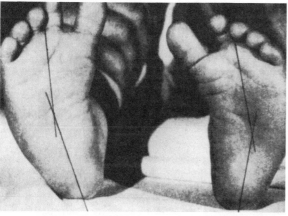

(From Behrman, R. E. (ed.): Nelson Textbook of Pediatrics, 14th ed. Philadelphia, W. B. Saunders Company, 1991; p. 1695; reprinted with permission.)

1. This picture shows (choose one)

(a) vertical talus
(b) metatarsus varus
(c) valgus deformity of the metatarsals
(d) clubfoot
(e) syndactyly

2. Which is the best initial treatment for this condition? (Assume the acute angle formed to be less than 20 degrees and the patient to be 2 weeks old.)

(a) Special shoes
(b) Stretching exercises
(c) Splinting
(d) Casting
(e) Surgery

3. Component(s) of clubfoot include (choose one or more)

(a) ankle equinus
(b) subtalar joint varus
(c) vertical varus
(d) varus deformity of the calcaneus
(e) valgus deformity of the metatarsals

4. Treatment for clubfoot usually includes (choose one or more)

(a) bedrest
(b) anti-inflammatory drugs
(c) manipulation (stretching exercises)
(d) casting
(e) early surgery

5. Which of the following is the most severe form of flatfoot?

(a) Vertical talus
(b) Talus-calcaneus coalition
(c) Calcaneus-navicular coalition
(d) Talonavicular coalition
(e) Peroneal spastic flatfoot

6. Usual treatment for mild to moderate flexible flat foot includes (choose one or more)

(a) reassurance
(b) "Thomas heel"
(c) stretching exercises
(d) casting
(e) surgery

7. Common reasons for "in-toeing" in toddlers include (choose one or more)

(a) calcaneovalgus
(b) metatarsus varus
(c) medial tibial torsion
(d) medial femoral torsion
(e) lateral femoral anteversion

8. The best treatment for "in-toeing" in toddlers is

(a) stretching exercises
(b) "orthopedic" shoes
(c) splints or casts
(d) surgery
(e) none of the above

9. Which of the following statements about shoes is/are correct?

(a) The purpose of shoes is to provide support for normal development of the bones
(b) Sneakers should not be worn until the child is over 2 years of age
(c) High-top shoes should be worn until the age of 2
(d) Soft-soled shoes should be the first shoes an infant wears
(e) "Orthopedic" shoes (with heel wedges, toe wedges, or both) should be prescribed for children with "out-toeing"

10. Which is the best initial treatment for dislocated, unrelocatable, congenitally dysplastic hips first discovered at 7 months of age?

(a) Triple diapers
(b) von Rosen splint or other rigid device
(c) Plaster spica case
(d) Traction
(e) Open (surgical) reduction

11. The most common cause of hip pain in infants and toddlers is

(a) dislocation
(b) infection
(c) transient synovitis ("toxic synovitis")
(d) leukemia
(e) juvenile rheumatoid arthritis

12. An overweight adolescent boy complains of pain in the medial aspect of his knee. He denies trauma, and he has not had a fever. The most likely diagnosis is

(a) toxic synovitis
(b) Legg-Calvé-Perthes disease
(c) medial collateral ligament (knee) strain
(d) slipped capital femoral epiphysis
(e) avulsion of the gastrocnemius muscle

QUESTIONS 13–14

An adolescent girl who is a cheerleader comes to you with a painful bump below her right knee. She denies fever or trauma.

13. Which is the most likely diagnosis?

(a) Legg-Calvé-Perthes disease
(b) Osteoid osteoma
(c) Osgood-Schlatter disease
(d) Osteochondritis dissicans
(e) Osteomyelitis of the tibial tubercle

14. The best treatment for this patient is

(a) decreased activity involving the knee
(b) anti-inflammatory drugs
(c) antibiotics
(d) excisional biopsy
(e) casting for 6 to 8 weeks

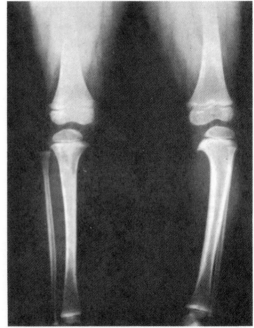

(From Behrman, R. E. (ed.): Nelson Textbook of Pediatrics, 14th ed. Philadelphia, W. B. Saunders Company, 1991; p. 1701; reprinted with permission.)

15. Which statement applies to the roentgen-ogram shown on p. 112 (lower right)? (Choose one.)

   (a) It demonstrates "bowleg"
   (b) Genu valgum is present
   (c) There is abnormal calcification of the lower tibias
   (d) The proximal end of the left tibia is abnormal
   (e) The legs are normal

16. Which of the following is/are *always* abnormal? (Choose one or more.)

   (a) Kyphosis
   (b) Lordosis
   (c) Scoliosis
   (d) Kyphoscoliosis
   (e) "Round shoulders"

17. Which form of scoliosis is more prevalent?

   (a) Postural
   (b) Functional
   (c) Neuromuscular
   (d) Congenital
   (e) Idiopathic

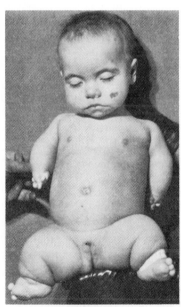

(From Behrman, R. E., and Vaughan, V. C. (eds.): Nelson Textbook of Pediatrics, 13th ed. Philadelphia, W. B. Saunders Company, 1987; p. 1355; reprinted with permission.)

18. The child's anomaly pictured above was most likely the result of

   (a) congenital infection
   (b) genetic mutation

   (c) maternal drug ingestion
   (d) birth trauma
   (e) unknown causes

QUESTIONS 19–20

A 2-year-old child is brought to you because he refuses to use his right arm. Any attempt to touch it is met with a cry, and the child will not hold objects in the right hand. The mother denies trauma, but she did pull the child by the arm recently when he refused to go into an elevator

19. The most likely diagnosis is

   (a) nonaccidental trauma (child abuse)
   (b) fracture of the radius
   (c) muscle strain of the right pronator
   (d) dislocated radial head
   (e) osteomyelitis

20. Plans for this child should include (choose one or more)

   (a) roentgenogram of the arm, then casting or splinting
   (b) supination of the forearm
   (c) antibiotics and splinting
   (d) alert the parents to the cause of the problem
   (e) report the case to a child welfare agency

21. Traumatic injury to the shoulder through overuse is most common in which of the following? (Choose one or more.)

   (a) Ballet
   (b) Swimming
   (c) Football
   (d) Baseball
   (e) Gymnastics

QUESTIONS 22–25

For each statement, select the appropriate Salter-Harris class(es) of epiphyseal fractures as

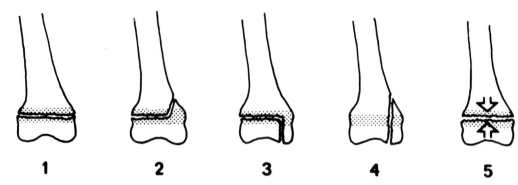

(From Behrman, R. E. (ed.): Nelson Textbook of Pediatrics, 14th ed. Philadelphia, W. B. Saunders Company, 1991; p. 1722; reprinted with permission.)

shown on the diagram above. Note: Each fracture type may be the answer to one, more than one, or none of the questions.

22. _____ The *two* most common
23. _____ Most often requires surgical treatment
24. _____ The *two* with the highest risk for growth disturbances
25. _____ Most difficult to diagnosis by roentgenogram

---

26. Blue sclerae are associated with which one of the following?

    (a) Chondrodystrophic calcificans congenita
    (b) Osteogenesis imperfecta
    (c) Thanatophoric dwarfism
    (d) Achondroplasia
    (e) Metatrophic dwarfism

27. Which of the following statements about achondroplastic dwarfism is/are true? (Choose one or more.)

    (a) It is an autosomal dominant trait
    (b) It results in marked shortening of the distal extremities
    (c) Neurologic complications are rare in infancy
    (d) Intelligence is usually normal
    (e) Roentgenograms of the bones show demineralization

28. A 6-month-old infant has fever, irritability, and swelling of the mandible. Laboratory studies show anemia and an elevated erythrocyte sedimenation rate. What is the most likely diagnosis?

    (a) Osteomyelitis
    (b) Rickets
    (c) Hypervitaminosis A
    (d) Chondrodysplasia punctata
    (e) Infantile cortical hyperostosis

29 Which of the following skeletal dysplasias is/are associated with hearing loss due to progressive eighth nerve encroachment? (Choose one or more.)

    (a) Kneist dysplasia
    (b) Osteopetrosis
    (c) Craniometaphyseal dysplasia
    (d) Hyperphosphatasia
    (e) Diastrophic dysplasia

30. Transient neonatal lesions that require no therapy include which of the following? (Choose one or more.)

    (a) Sebaceous hyperplasia
    (b) Milia
    (c) Salmon patch
    (d) Erythema toxicum
    (e) Mongolian spots

31. Steroids are effective in treating which of the following? (Choose one or more.)

    (a) Nevus flammeus
    (b) Capillary hemangioma
    (c) Cavernous hemangioma
    (d) Blue rubber bleb nevus
    (e) Spider angiomas

32. Which of the following is/are associated with predisposition for malignant melanoma?

    (a) Nevus of Ota
    (b) Giant hairy nevus

(c) Comedone nevi
(d) Nevus sebaceus
(e) Achromic nevi

33. Which of the following statements regarding erythema multiforme is/are correct?

(a) The vesicles are infectious
(b) There are multiple causes
(c) Marked pruritus is a feature of the disorder
(d) Iris or target lesions are pathognomonic
(e) Corticosteroid cream is the treatment of choice

QUESTIONS 34–39

For each of the following dermatologic disorders, select the most likely site of vesicle formation (a–e).

34. _____ Toxic epidermal necrolysis   (a) Granular layer
35. _____ Staphylococcal scalded skin syndrome   (b) Intracorneal layer
36. _____ Erythema multiforme   (c) Intraepidermal layer
37. _____ Bullous impetigo   (d) Subcorneal layer
38. _____ Candidiasis   (e) Subepidermal layer
39. _____ Viral blisters

40. Causes of allergic contact dermatitis include which of the following? (Choose one or more.)

(a) Nickel
(b) Thimerosal (Merthiolate)
(c) Neomycin
(d) Topical antihistamines
(e) Topical anesthetics

41. Hypopigmented, round, macular, slightly scaly lesions that have a poorly marginated border and do not itch are characistic of which one of the following?

(a) Candidiasis
(b) Pityriasis alba
(c) Pityriasis rosea
(d) Lichen simplex chronicus
(e) Dyshidrotic eczema

42. Which of the following is/are true of seborrheic dermatitis? (Choose one or more.)

(a) It is most common in infants
(b) It is also known as cradle cap
(c) It can be reactivated by stress
(d) Topical corticosteroid preparations usually control the lesions
(e) An intractable form of the disorder is associated with a functional disorder of the fifth component of complement

43. Which of the following is/are associated with increased photosensitivity? (Choose one or more.)

(a) Tetracyclines
(b) Sulfonamides
(c) Herpes simplex
(d) Erythropoietic protoporphyria
(e) Lichen simplex chronicus

44. Which one of the following begins with a "herald patch" and has a "Christmas tree" distribution?

(a) Guttate psoriasis
(b) Lichen spinulosus
(c) Keratosis pilaris
(d) Xeroderma pigmentosum
(e) Pityriasis rosea

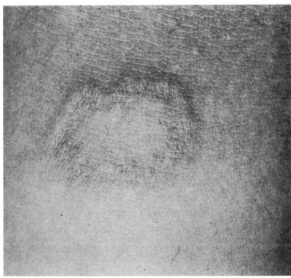

(From Behrman, R. E. (eds): Nelson Textbook of Pediatrics, 14th ed. Philadelphia, W. B. Saunders Company, 1991; p. 1659; reprinted with permission.)

45. The lesion shown above is raised, firm, and not pruitic. It is most commonly found on the dorsum of the hands and feet. What is it?

(a) Erythema marginatum

(b) Tinea corporis
(c) Granuloma annulare
(d) Erythema multiforme
(e) Papular urticaria

(a) Mucoceles
(b) Lip pits
(c) Aphthous stomatitis
(d) Primary herpes stomatitis
(e) Fordyce disease

QUESTIONS 46–48

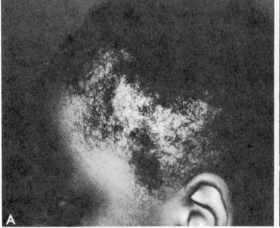
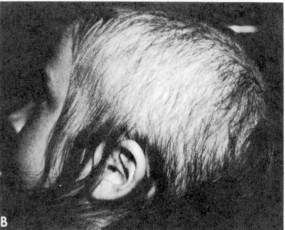
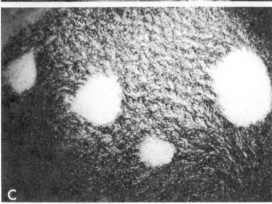

(From Behrman, R. E. (ed.): Nelson Textbook of Pediatrics, 14th ed. Philadelphia, W. B. Saunders Company, 1991; p. 1667; reprinted with permission.)

For each figure above, select the correct diagnosis (a–e).

46. _____ Photograph A
47. _____ Photograph B
48. _____ Photograph C

(a) Traction alopecia
(b) Toxic alopecia
(c) Trichotillomania
(d) Alopecia areata
(e) Alopecia totalis

49. Recurrent erythematous papules that progress to necrotic ulcers on the labial, buccal, and lingual mucosa are characteristic of which one of the following?

QUESTIONS 50–54

For each of the following conditions, select the associated organism (a–d).

50. _____ Ecthyma
51. _____ Folliculitis
52. _____ Ritter disease
53. _____ "Swimming pool" granuloma
54. _____ Blistering distal dactylitis

(a) Group A β-hemolytic streptococci
(b) *Staphylococcus aureus*
(c) Atypical mycobacteria
(d) Fungi

55. Cutaneous fungal infections caused by which of the following organisms show fluores-

cence with a Wood lamp? (Choose one or more.)

(a) *Pityrosporum orbiculare*
(b) *Microsporum audouinii*
(c) *Trichophyton tonsurans*
(d) *Trichophyton rubrum*
(e) *Candida albicans*

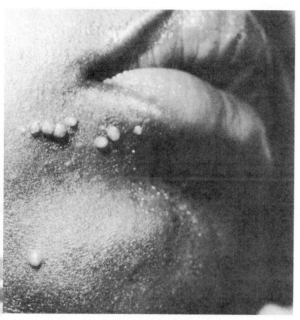

(From Behrman, R. E. (ed.): Nelson Textbook of Pediatrics, 14th ed. Philadelphia, W. B. Saunders Company, 1991; p. 1679; reprinted with permission.)

56. The lesions shown above have been present for three months. What is the diagnosis?

(a) Verrucous warts
(b) Condylomata acuminata
(c) Herpes simplex
(d) Varicella zoster
(e) Molluscum contagiosum

QUESTIONS 57–58

Questions 57–58 refer to the following figures (*A*, *B*, and *C*) on p. 118:

57. The disorder shown in A and B is

(a) papular urticaria
(b) multiple insect bites

(c) scabies
(d) pediculosis
(e) Rocky Mountain spotted fever

58. The causative organism shown in C is a

(a) mite
(b) tick
(c) louse
(d) chigger
(e) insect

---

59. Important factors in the pathogenesis and treatment of acne include (choose one or more)

(a) diet
(b) climate
(c) control of surface bacteria
(d) topical vitamin A acid
(e) systemic tetracycline

QUESTIONS 60–64

For each of the following conditions, select the appropriate treatment(s) (a–e). (One or more treatment may be correct for each condition.)

60. _____ Impetigo   (a) Wet dressing
61. _____ Seborrheic   (b) Bath oil
            dermatitis   (c) Keratolytic agents
62. _____ Dry skin   (d) Tar compounds
63. _____ Ichthyosis   (e) Sulfur shampoos
64. _____ Psoriasis

---

65. Which of the following statements regarding the use of topical corticosteroids is/are correct? (Choose one or more.)

(a) They should be applied in a very thin film
(b) Lotions are better absorbed than ointments
(c) Occlusive wraps enhance their percutaneous absorption
(d) Fluorinated corticosteroids are most effective in young infants
(e) Adverse effects include striae, atrophy, and hypopigmentation

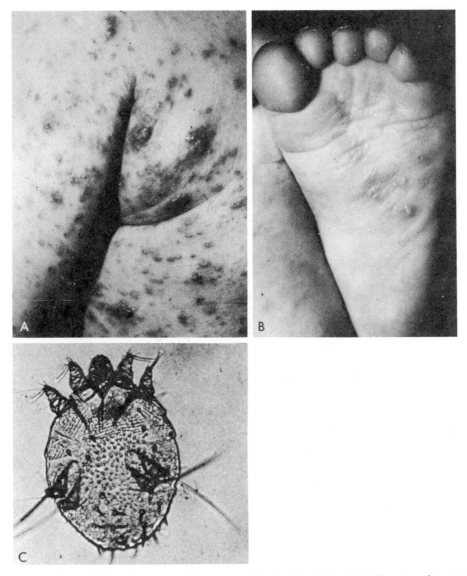

(From Behrman, R. E. (ed.): Nelson Textbook of Pediatrics, 14th ed. Philadelphia, W. B. Saunders Company, 1991; p. 1681; reprinted with permission.)

23

Unclassified Diseases and Environmental Health Hazards

This potpourri of subjects will almost finish us off. As often happens when you try to review a broad subject, at the end there are a number of items left that do not comfortably fit into any of the previous sections. It may be a sign of progress that there are fewer entities left over for this chapter in this edition of the textbook than there were a decade ago. The fact that SIDS and poisoning occur at the end of the book in no way diminishes their importance (although the same may not be true for amyloidosis and progeria).

In any event, the knowledge that the end of this multiple choice marathon is in sight should spur you on in spite of the conglomerate nature of the material.

1. Which of the following statements is/are true of the sudden infant death syndrome (SIDS)?

   (a) The mechanism of death is sudden ventricular fibrillation
   (b) The incidence of the syndrome is increasing yearly
   (c) The ability to identify "vulnerable" children is a significant advance since parents can now try to prevent the syndrome
   (d) Autopsy is necessary to establish the diagnosis
   (e) Many cases of SIDS are actually child abuse

QUESTIONS 2–5

For each of the following findings, select the assocaited disease (a–d).

2. _____ Painless, boggy synovial effusions of tendon sheaths
3. _____ Eosinophilic granuloma of bone
4. _____ Renal amyloidosis
5. _____ Atherosclerosis

   (a) Schüller-Christian syndrome
   (b) Familial Mediterranean fever
   (c) Sarcoidosis
   (d) Progeria

6. Which of the following is/are true about radiation injury?

   (a) Beta irradiation causes biochemical damage, while gamma radiation is biophysically damaging
   (b) The greater the differentiation of cells, the more sensitive they are to radiation injury
   (c) Early signs of radiation injury include leukopenia and thrombocytopenia
   (d) In utero exposure to diagnostic radiation causes a 50% increase in the likelihood of death by cancer before age 10
   (e) Chromosomal abnormalities are still found in the peripheral lymphocytes of the Hiroshima atomic bomb survivors

QUESTIONS 7–10

For each set of symptoms, select the associated etiologic agent or food (a–e).

7. _____ Vomiting and abdominal cramps 4 hours after eating potato salad
8. _____ Bloody diarrhea 48 to 72 hours after

   (a) *Salmonella* species
   (b) Staphylococcal enterotoxin
   (c) *Clostridium botulinum* toxin
   (d) *Gonyaulax catanella*

eating sausage   (e) *Amanita*
9. _____ Parasthesias,   *muscaria*
burning of the
tongue,
numbness of
the face
10. _____ Salivation,
sweating, ab-
dominal pain

11. Children who are suspected of having ingested chemical or drug poisons should be
given syrup of ipecac UNLESS (choose one
or more)

(a) they are comatose
(b) the ingested agent is alkali
(c) it has been 4 hours since the ingestion
of salicylate
(d) the drug ingested is unknown
(e) activated charcoal is available

12. Urine acidification is contraindicated in the
treatment of poisoning by which of the following agents? (Choose one or more.)

(a) Salicylates
(b) Amphetamines
(c) Phencyclidine
(d) Mercury
(e) Iron

13. Which of the following is/are true about
acetaminophen toxicity?

(a) All age groups are affected
(b) Hepatic toxicity is the major problem
(c) Plasma drug levels obtained 10 hours
after ingestion are *not* of therapeutic
importance
(d) *N*-acetyl-L-cysteine is of therapeutic
value if given within 24 hours
(e) Hemodialysis will reverse hepatic toxicity

14. Which of the following is/are true of salicylism?

(a) It involves direct stimulation of the respiratory center of the brain
(b) The presence of salicylates in the plasma
causes a profound metabolic alkalosis
(c) Significant bleeding occurs as a result
of gastrointestinal irritation and is a major problem in acute salicylism
(d) Nonionized salicylate in the urine is
rapidly excreted

(e) Phenistix turn brown to purple in salicylism

15. True statements about barbiturate poisoning include (choose one or more)

(a) It is the most common type of poisoning
in adolescents
(b) The primary effect is depression of the
central nervous system
(c) Alkalinization of the urine increases the
excretion rate of short-acting barbiturates
(d) A flat electroencephalogram and fixed,
dilated pupils indicate brain death in a
patient with barbiturate poisoning
(e) Peritoneal dialysis is more effective than
alkalinization of the urine in treating
poisoning with long-acting barbiturates

16. True statements about hydrocarbon poisoning include (choose one or more)

(a) Low viscosity hydrocarbons are less
likely to cause problems than those of
high viscosity
(b) The pathologic findings are similar to
those seen in acute hemorrhagic edema
and bronchopneumonia
(c) Emesis and lavage are indicated in alert
patients with large ingestions
(d) Systemic corticosteroids are indicated
to reduce inflammation
(e) Fever and leukocytosis indicate secondary bacterial infection

17. Which of the following statements regarding iron poisoning in childern is/are correct?

(a) The primary manifestation is gastric irritation
(b) A low serum iron level 18 hours after
ingestion indicates a good prognosis
(c) Normal-colored urine following injection of 1 gram of deferoxamine is reassuring
(d) Initial treatment should include emesis
and lavage with deferoxamine solution
(e) Deferoxamine should be continued until the urine is clear for 24 hours

QUESTIONS 18–20

A 7-year-old boy who has been under treatment for enuresis suddenly develops agitation,
confusion, and hallucinations 1 hour after going

to bed. His mother had given him one pill before bed, but when questioned, she found the bottle to be empty. (There were at least 15 pills.)

18. The most likely toxic drug in this case is

(a) a heavy metal
(b) a salicylate
(c) a barbiturate
(d) a tricyclic antidepressant
(e) an amphetamine

19. Initial treatment for this child should include (choose one or more)

(a) emesis
(b) lavage with a chelating agent
(c) administration of activated charcoal
(d) forced diuresis
(e) alkalinization of the urine

20. Which of the following has/have usefulness in the treatment of this child?

(a) British antilewisite
(b) Penicillamine
(c) Physostigmine
(d) Propranolol
(e) Sodium bicarbonate

---

21. Which of the following plants is responsible for most reports to poison centers? (Choose one.)

(a) Jimson weed
(b) Poinsettia
(c) Philodendrom
(d) Pokeweed
(e) Holly

22. A pink color of the hands and feet associated with listlessness and hypotonia is most likely to be caused by

(a) acute inorganic mercury poisoning
(b) chronic inorganic mercury poisoning
(c) chronic organic mercury poisoning
(d) polychlorinated biphenyl (PCB) ingestion
(e) lead poisoning

23. The principal manifestations of lead poisoning include (choose one or more)

(a) microcytic hypochromic anemia
(b) rash
(c) peripheral neuropathy

(d) colic
(e) encephalopathy

24. Which of the following is/are found in children with lead poisoning?

(a) Increased erythrocyte δ-aminolevulinate dehydratase
(b) Increased urinary δ-aminolevulinic acid
(c) Decreased urinary coproporphyrin
(d) Decreased urinary uroporphyrin
(e) Increased free erythrocyte protoporphyrin

25. Treatment of category II lead poisoning should include (choose one or more)

(a) environmental control
(b) chelation with British antilewisite (intramuscular)
(c) chelation with CaEDTA (intramuscular)
(d) zinc supplementation (oral)
(e) D-penicillamine (oral)

26. Chemicals that have been associated with birth defects in human infants include which of the following? (Choose one or more.)

(a) Methylmercury
(b) Polychlorinated biphenyl (PCB)
(c) Dioxin
(d) Cigarette smoke
(e) Diethylstilbestrol

27. Which of the following statements about chemical pollutants is/are true?

(a) The presence of polychlorinated biphenyl (PCB) in breast milk is an indication for cessation of breast feeding
(b) Asbestos fibers in water have been linked to mesothelioma in children
(c) Increased mortality from lung cancer has been demonstrated among persons living near arsenic-emitting smelters
(d) Air pollution (sulfur oxides, carbon monoxide, ozone) has been associated with an increased incidence of respiratory disease
(e) Food preservatives have been demonstrated to increase hyperactivity in children

28. Antivenins are available for bites or stings of which of the following? (Choose one or more.)

(a) Rattlesnake
(b) Stonefish
(c) Gila monster
(d) Portuguese man-of-war
(e) Stingray

29. The most common complication of dog bite in the United States is

(a) Strep or staph infection
(b) *Pasteurella multocida* infection
(c) Rabies
(d) Tetanus
(e) Psychological disturbances

30. Each of the following has a venom causing toxic reactions in humans EXCEPT

(a) Black widow spider
(b) Brown recluse spider
(c) Tarantula
(d) Scorpion

Answers

1

The Field of Pediatrics

1. (c) Astrologic charts are widely published but credible data are lacking as to their influence on child health. (*p. 1*)

2. (e) Although there have been significant gains in reducing the neonatal mortality rate, these gains are still much less than those in the postneonatal period. This trend reflects the significant impact of immunization and sanitation and the effects of antibiotics on acute infectious disease. (*p. 1*)

3. (a) Nationally, 24% of children (<18 years) lived with one parent—88% of them with their mother, so (b) is true. (c) and (d) are true, true and related as to cause and effect. (*p. 2*)

4. (d) The birthrate has risen and the adolescent population has declined over the last decade, so (a) and (b) are false. The *number* of children has increased annually (although their *percentage* has decreased, so (c) is false also. (*p. 2*)

5. (d) Accidents, homicide, and suicide—conditions for which we have no vaccine—are the major killers of children. The mortality rate does fall after the first year but climbs again in adolescence. (*p. 2*)

6. (c) Diagnosis-related groups (DRGs) are the latest in a long series of federal efforts to restrain medical cost inflation, which was fueled intensely in the 1970s by increases in costly technology, and the third-party insuror/fee-for-service system. Peer review may have improved quality, and may have improved utilization, but nothing has yet reduced costs significantly. (*p. 4*)

7. (c) Anyone answering (a) or (b) needs to reevaluate what the role of a health provider is. Knowing it all, even *if* one had the cortical ability to do so, is not enough. Cognitive knowledge is only a part of what we need. A cynic I know once pointed out (for those of you who answered [d]) that subspecialization is the process of learning more and more about less and less, until you know everything about nothing. (*p. 4*)

2
Ethical and Cultural Issues in Pediatrics

1. **(c)** Paternalism (the next edition might say "parentalism") is generally the responsibility of parents. Physicians use this principle to overcome parental objections when the outcome is judged to be for the benefit of the child. Autonomy (a) is also involved in these cases. (*p. 6*)

2. **(d)** There is rarely a circumstance in which the physician should not tell the truth. It is particularly important in relationships where one person (the physician) is in a powerful position of trust. (*p. 6*)

3. **(b)** Few disagree that children should participate in their health care decisions, but they must be developmentally and cognitively competent to do so. (*p. 6*)

4. **(e)** The principle of confidentiality of the physician-patient relationship is crucial, but there are clear exceptions when the information discloses a situation that is harmful to others. (*p. 6*)

5. **(f)** Physicians may find themselves in situations in which the best interests of the child and family conflict. Intrafamilial abuse, "Baby Doe" situations, and contraceptive use by adolescents are some examples. (*p. 6*)

6. **(c)** Although discarded newborns do get the "Baby Doe" label, the legal issue referred to was brought to light subsequent to the death of an infant born with Down syndrome and esophageal atresia who was provided no care and allowed to die at 6 days of age. (*p. 7*)

7. **(e)** Although some individuals may believe they have all five qualities needed to make ethical decisions, few do. To ensure the best decisions, a collaborative process using review boards has been developed in most communities. (*p. 7*)

8. **(b)** Although there were early problems in PKU screening (because of lack of certainty about the significance of mildly elevated levels), this screening program is on solid ground. Others require more analysis, among them those listed in the question require more study (e.g., cystic fibrosis, HIV). (*p. 8*)

9. **(c)** Innovative therapy is associated with the least protection for children with or without informed consent. Since there is no intent to gather information, protocols are not peer-reviewed and potential toxicity or adverse reaction is not systematically assessed. (*p. 9*)

10. **(d)** There is little benefit of doing a C-section by court order when the likelihood of survival of a 26-week fetus is so small, so this dilemma is the least difficult of those presented. The other three situations confront us often in clinical practice and the risk-to-benefit ratio or ethical dilemmas of each are much narrower. (*p. 9*)

11. **(a)** Residence in an ethnic enclave will *decrease* acculturation. Other factors positively correlated in addition to those listed in (b), (c), and (d) are: second generation or greater in host cultural area, less contact with ethnic area of origin, and less contact with extended family, (*p. 10*)

12. **(c)** Recognizing cultural practices, accepting them (as long as they are not hazardous to the child's health), and incorporating them into traditional medicine will be associated with the best outcomes. (*p. 10*)

13. **(b)** Empacho is gastroenteritis and responds to teas. (*p. 10*)

14. **(c)** Mal (de) ojo—the evil eye—will be addressed by benediction. (*p. 11*)

15. **(a)** Caida de mollera—sunken fontanelle—is a result of significant dehydration. (*p. 11*)

3

Growth and Development

1. (b) Physical growth and development are *not* constant, and emotional growth and development begin in the newborn period. (d) is only partly true—heredity has a lot to do with the process. (*p. 13*)

2. (c) In an ideal (mesokurtic) curve, all of these values are the same. When the curves are skewed the median value is most representative. (*p. 13*)

3. (b); 4. (c); 5. (a) The main point to be made in this series of questions is that a single measurement on a growth chart does not make a diagnosis. Those of you who started with (a) should review the basic science years; if you started with (c) you probably spent too much time there; (d) would have given you the same data (and most junior students on their first rotation wouldn't have the nerve to ask).

To make a simple additional point, birth weight and height are usually remembered and always recorded, and whether the infant was pre-term or term is also a key. An infant under the third percentile can actually be between the 10th and 25th percentiles when appropriate adjustments are made for gestational age.

6. (b) Organogenesis is a first-trimester function. In the second, the fetus grows in length and organ function develops. The other statements are correct. (*pp. 14–15*)

7. (d) All of these increase the risks of adverse growth and development, but an acute episode of malnutrition in an otherwise healthy woman will cause less damage than the other choices given. (*p. 15*)

8. (a) Respiratory movements begin at 18 weeks, and the tidal flow of amniotic fluid contributes to pulmonary arborization. Respiratory efforts outside the uterus are generally not successful until 24 to 26 weeks, or later. (*pp. 14–15*)

9. (e) Newborn infants have a decreased ability to concentrate urine. (*p. 16*)

10. (a) A low hemoglobin in a newborn should make you worry about whether there has been hemorrhage, hemolysis, or failure to make red cells in utero. A low neutrophil count should make you worry about sepsis. (*p. 16*)

11. (b) Newborns have been shown to fixate visually during the quiet alert state. This state represents 10% of a 24-hour day. (*pp. 17–18*)

12. (b) We are indebted to Drs. Brazleton and Prechtl and others for teaching us how to understand the complex behavior of newborns. See Question 11.

13. (e) This is a throwaway as far as being a tough question, and the Board of Examiners would groan at the sight of an "all of the above—none of the above" question. I threw it in, though, because there is an important point to be made. For years mothers would come to us at two-week visits and say, "When can babies see?" "Six to eight weeks," we would answer confidently. What they were really saying was, "My baby looks at me," but we wouldn't accept it. Now we know that newborns can see and hear and are very sophisticated indeed; so, don't pass off those neonatal smiles as "gas." (*pp. 17–18*)

14. (c) Premature infants have more developmental problems than their term counterparts at the same gestational age. The effects of infection and anoxia are of etiologic importance here, as well as impaired (or at least more difficult) parent-infant attachment. (*p. 18*)

15. (N) Infants lose up to 10% or so of their birth weight, then gain 25 to 30 grams a day. Therefore, returning to birth weight in 7 to 10 days is normal. (*p. 16*)

16. (N) Most infants get teeth earlier, but edentulous 1-year-olds are neither rare nor of concern. (*p. 19*)

17. (N) The anterior fontanelle can enlarge before it decreases in size. (*p. 18*)

18. (C) Not smiling responsively at 10 weeks is worrisome. (*p. 19*)

19. (N) Not worrisome yet. (*p. 20*)

20. (N) Classic behavior coincident with separation anxiety. (*p. 21*)

21. (N) Appetites become variable in the second year. (*p. 21*)

22. (N) Again, a classic behavior for a 4-year-old. (*p. 26*)

23. (N) Lack of speech intelligibility is not abnormal until well into the third year. (*pp. 21, 26*)

24. (N) Few issues generate as much debate as toilet training. In the 1940s and 1950s the answer would have been (c), since pediatricians recommend "training" at 8 to 12 months. Times change, cultures change, and we've changed too. It is okay for a 2½-year-old to wear diapers. (*p. 21*)

25. (c) Waking up at night (if, in fact, the baby has already slept through the night) at 6 to 8 months is common behavior. Whether this is related to separation anxiety or something else (teething?) is not clear (edentulous babies wake up, too). (a) would be highly unlikely, since 6½-month-old boys who have grown normally almost never get urinary tract infections. (b) would be unnecessary and would probably lead to hunger and a fussier baby. (d) is wrong because DTP reactions occur 4 to 36 hours after the shot, not 2 weeks. (*p. 21*)

26. (d) Molars erupt at 18 months, 3 years, 6 years, 14 years, and 18 to 20 years. The 6-year molars are the first permanent teeth. (*p. 27*)

27. (a) The relative macrocephaly of infants has been recognized by shirtmakers for years, which is why there are snaps in the shoulder seam. (*p. 16, Fig. 3–2*)

28. (e) The second year of infancy is very imitative. In the third year the child begins the independent "no" stage. The loss of appetite is a logical consequence of the deceleration in growth. (*p. 21*)

29. (a) There is nothing like school to promote infections in children. (b) would not be incorrect but would be expensive and probably unnecessary in a child who has grown and developed normally for 5 years. (c), (d), and (e) would be unjustified. (*p. 27*)

30. (d) No comment needed. (*pp. 28–32*)

31. (SMR 1); 32. (SMR 2); 33. (SMR 5); 34. (SMR 4); 35. (SMR 2) (*pp. 29–30*)

36. (b); 37. (c) The relationship of SMR to growth, strength, hematocrit, etc. is important. A neighbor of mine put it simply: children in the 12- to 15-year-old age group should not be classed by chronologic age, but whether they are "hairs" or "bares." (*pp. 28–30*)

38. (c) SMR ratings have little to do with academic performance, but they are now clearly related to biochemical and endocrine changes in adolescents. (*p. 39*)

39. (b) Physical separation is not necessary *during* adolescence; it is desirable after adolescence. (*pp. 49–50*) See also Chapter 10.

40. (d) All of the other choices reflect occasional adolescent states of mind, but the George Allen "the future is now" attitude is all pervasive. (*pp. 49–50*)

41. (b) Most relationships in early adolescence are same sex and relatively superficial. The other statements are true. (*pp. 49–50*)

42. (b) Kohlberg's work involved moral development. Freud and Fraiberg focused on different subjects or stages. Domain-specific knowledge is the second of seven discrete stages of cognitive development as described by Piaget. (*p. 30*)

43. (b) Ossification of the clavicles *and* the distal femoral and proximal tibial epiphyses are all present at birth. Girls are less variable in bone development than boys at all ages, but especially in late adolescence. (*p. 37*)

44. (c) Newborns do not have the enzymes necessary to metabolize sulfonamides, so (a) is incorrect. (c) is wrong as the cytochrome P450 *is* affected by androgens but is not involved in sulfonamide metabolism. (d) is also incorrect. ADHD is not linked to sulfonamide metabolism. (*p. 39*)

45–46. This edition of the textbook eliminates a long discussion of the DDST. Since I am from Denver, however, and had early bonding to this test (my children being early research subjects), I left them in.

47. (b); 48. (d); 49. (a); 50. (c) Each of these men contributed greatly to our understanding of child development theory, building on each others' work. (*pp. 43–45*)

51. (e) The "difficult" child was most at risk for subsequent behavioral problems in childhood in Chess and Thomas' study. Even "easy" children had problems, though, if the child's and parents' temperaments didn't fit. (*p. 46*)

52. (e) "Other" is right—all of the above or none of the above might be appropriate as well. The best time for parents to have the next child is when they are ready. (*p. 47*)

53. (b) Teleologically, if it weren't for these two developmental stages, parents would never want children to leave home. (*pp. 46–49*)

54. (d) Parents should not use punishment of their children as an emotional release. It should also be said that whereas consistency is universally prescribed, it is probably overwhelmingly inhuman. (*pp. 47–48*)

55. (a) Progressive demyelinating disease, though possible, is a very unlikely cause of school problems. The rest are common. (*p. 48*)

56. (d) 80% of 19-year-old boys; 60% of 19-year-old girls. The last edition pointed out that 44% of 13- to 15-year-old boys had experienced intercourse. (*pp. 32, 49*)

57. (a) Early emancipation tends to increased anxiety in the adolescent. The other answers are reasonable, if not entirely easy, things to do. (*p. 50*)

58. (a) Identity and moral development are characteristics of middle and early adolescence. Depression often can be seen but is not characteristic. (*p. 32*)

59. (c) Remembering 6 forward and 5 backward digits is appropriate for an 11- to 12 + -year-old. The other tasks are 4–5 year-old milestones. (*p. 42*)

60. (a) The expressive language behavior of beginning to mimic sounds occurs at 40 weeks of age—which is the time infants develop the receptive language behavior of responding to their own name. (*p. 41*)

61. (e) is most likely, even though we sometimes have the tendency to blame allergy or viruses for everything. (*p. 59*)

62. (b) Most 2-year-olds make their parents pay for leaving them by ignoring them on their return. (*p. 59*)

63. (c); 64. (b) Denial is first, guilt later. Children should neither be sheltered from nor overly involved in funerals and other rituals at 5 years of age or older. (*pp. 51–52*)

65. (c) States have passed laws requiring permanency planning to reduce the tendency for foster children (most already abused and neglected) to "drift" from placement to placement. (*p. 51*)

66. (c) This question requires a careful reading of the Wallerstein and Kelly data. It is 45% of children who were "doing well" after 10 years, not 60 to 70%. (*p. 52*)

67. (c) The actual figure is 30 to 40 hours weekly. (*p. 53*)

68. (a) It is the toddlers who have tantrums. (*p. 56*)

69. (c) Psychiatric disturbances are more common in brain-injured children, as they are in epileptics. (*p. 57*)

70. (b) It is voluntary musculature or organs of special senses that are targets for conversion reactions (e.g., blindness, paralysis, etc.). (*p. 57*)

71. (d) These children are often hyperactive. (*p. 57*)

72. (d) The activity level is often normal in patients with anorexia nervosa. (*p. 533*)

73. (c) There are few calories in dirt. (*p. 58*)

74. (c) This is an important statistic. I have long been depressed about our compulsion to have children clean and dry before they are physiologically able to be. Diurnal enuresis is not common in 5-year-olds, but neither does it require treatment with imipramine. (*p. 58*)

75. (b) Encopresis is much less common than enuresis and usually serves as a symptom of significant pathology. Although not mentioned in the text, I have personally seen encopresis as the presenting symptom of sexual abuse. (*p. 59*)

76. (e) Another "all of the above," but true. (*p. 59*)

77. (a) The belief that (b) is correct leads to repeated attempts to "break" children (a distressing term and concept), which probably has the effect of reinforcing the behavior. (*pp. 59–60*)

78. **(d)** Ignoring open masturbation in older children is not appropriate. One would again wonder about sexual abuse and should explore the possibility. (*p. 69*)

79. **(b)** Again, it isn't mentioned, but I believe that many suicide attempts are related to incest. Sexually abused children may be a significant part of those cases with "multiple problems" or "no information." (*pp. 63–64*)

80. **(c)** These episodes are harmless and should not be reinforced. (*p. 65*)

81. **(b)** Boys are significantly more often affected than girls. (*pp. 67–69*)

82. **(a)** Home and school visits should be done more often in general, but especially here. (*p. 68*)

83. **(a)** Structure before drug treatment is harder to do but better for many children. Hyperactivity untreated does not get better with time. (*pp. 68–69*)

84. **(e)** Dependency, either early or late in adolescence, does not seem to occur. (*p. 68*)

85. **(c)** It is the secretiveness that is worrisome. (*pp. 69–70*)

86. **(c)** The cause is not known, period. Parents should not be made to feel guilty. (*p. 71*)

87. **(d)** is false. Exhibitionism is common early (3 to 5 years) but decreases with age. The rest are true and common. (*pp. 70–71*)

88. **(a)** Often (c) is done, but obtaining more history never hurts.

89. **(c)** A discrepant history is a hallmark of abuse—whether it is bilateral skull fractures in an infant who rolled off the couch, *or*, as in this case, a rash that isn't there. (*p. 79*)

90. **(c)** Child abuse crosses all socioeconomic lines. Approximately 1% are physically abused, and at least that number are neglected. The number of deaths is approximate but too high! (*p. 79*)

91. **(b)** Less than 10% of abusive parents are psychotic; the incidence is *increased* in military populations; 80% of abusive parents can be helped although it gets tougher as resources shrink. (*pp. 79–81*)

92. **(e)** Physical findings are sometimes confirmatory but not often present and usually not diagnostic. Forensic studies should *always* be done if there is a history of ejaculation within 72 hours. Dolls, and drawings, are a useful adjunct to obtaining a history. The chlamydia slide test is too unreliable for diagnosis—cultures are better. (*p. 82*)

93. **(a)** These are "low-severity" handicaps but are increasingly being recognized. (*p. 84*)

94. **(a)** Narrative dysfluency is a linguistic disorder. (*p. 85*)

95. **(a)** Repeating the year may be necessary, but only if (b), (c), (d), and (e) are unsuccessful. Automatically leaving a child back may contribute to a "failure syndrome," which might exacerbate the problem. (*p. 89*)

96. **(d)** is correct. There are fewer chronic illnesses in adults, but more adults suffer from them. As technology advances, more chronic illness replaces death as an outcome. Families bear most of the cost (and stress) of caring for these children. (*p. 92*)

97. **(d)**; 98. **(b)**; 99. **(c)**; 100. **(a)** Table 3–26 will be helpful here. The evaluation of mentally retarded children—more appropriately called children with disabilities—is complex, but important for prognostic and therapeutic reasons. (*p. 97*)

4

Nutrition and Nutritional Disorders

1. (c) is true. (a) and (b) are both false. Water requirements of infants and adults are about equal per 100 calories, with infants having a greater per-kilogram requirement. Phototherapy increases water requirements by raising body temperature. (*p. 105*)

2. (b) The clinical assessment is the easiest. BMR calculations are difficult and not routinely available. (*p. 107*)

3. (b) The others are: leucine, isoleucine, phenylalanine, methionine, and histidine. (*p. 107*)

4. (b); 5. (e); 6. (a); 7. (c); 8. (c) These are fairly obvious. Amylase breaks starch down into simpler sugars. Disaccharidases digest disaccharides, of which lactose and maltose are two. Phosphorylase is an intracellular enzyme and not a correct answer here. (*pp. 107–109*)

9. (c) These are all synthesized by bacteria in the intestinal tract. (*pp. 113–114*)

10. (c) A trick question! Iron is *not* a trace element. (*p. 109*)

11. (a) Milk is a poor source of copper and iron. (*p. 110; Table 4–5*)

12. (c) Yeast is the anwer to this trivia question. (*p. 110*)

13. (c) Although crying infants *may* be hungry, the surest way to lead to overfeeding would be to suggest to mothers that food should be used to quiet a fussy, crying baby; (a) then is not true; (b) is only partly true. Many newborn infants will sleep for longer than 4 hours during one period a day, making up for lost time by feeding every 2 to 3 hours during another part of the day. (d) is recommended by some grandmothers, but never proven; it is not nutritionally sound. Breast milk and formula are both good sources of vitamin C; for an infant receiving evaporated milk, a vitamin supplement is simpler and more effective than juice. (*pp. 115–117*)

14. (C); 15. (A); 16. (C); 17. (A); 18. (B); 19. (A); 20. (A); 21. (B); 22. (A) The bottom line is that breast milk is for babies, and, except in unusual circumstances, cow's milk should be reserved for calves. (*pp. 116–122*)

23. (b) Breast-fed infants may have stools each day initially. As time goes on, the milk is so well utilized that little is left for stool formation, and infants may have as few as one soft stool every 7 to 10 days. The facts that the infant is not ill (is actively nursing) and is not dehydrated (10 to 12 wet diapers a day) make disease unlikely, so (d) would not be a good choice. Note that fever is *not* a good sign of disease in newborns (they get hypothermic when septic) so that bit of history was a red herring. (c) is wrong, since formulas and cereals are generally constipating. (*p. 128*)

24. (d) This is still a normal baby.

25–33 (*pp. 122–124*)

25. (D) Sweetened condensed milk is for baking, not drinking.

26. (B) The solute load of whole milk is too large for the newborn kidney.

27. (C) Newborns will need to have sugar syrup added and vitamin supplements, but evaporated milk is fine.

28. (B) Same reason as 26.

29. (C) For those allergic to cow's milk-based formulas.

30. (D) No nutritive value at all for growing infants or children.

31. (B) Same as 26. Also, growing infants need some fat.

32. (D) Should be reversed for obese children on a diet.

33. (D) Generally unsafe bacteriologically.

34. (c) Recent evidence shows that breast milk contains adequate amounts of vitamin D (water-soluble form), and manufacturers add vitamin D to their prepared formulas. (*p. 122*)

35. **(d)** Although breast milk contains relatively less iron by weight, the iron is more bio-available than the iron in cereals. Fruits, yellow vegetables, and cow's milk are poor sources of iron. (*p. 127*)

36. **(d)** Codeine appears in breast milk and is constipating. All the other choices may be causes of loose stools. (*p. 128*)

37. **(a)** Vegan mothers, who do not take B_{12} supplements, may have their infant develop methylmalonic acidemia. The other choices are either seen in vegan children or adults (c) and (d), or are more common in non-vegans (b) and (e). (*p. 130*)

38. **(a)** Most children will choose an adequate diet. I know of no normal children who have starved themselves to death. They grow less in the second year, get "picker," and actively seek power struggles with their parents. (*p. 129*)

39. **(c)** Kwashiorkor is primarily *protein* malnutrition. Marasmus is primarily caloric malnutrition. (*pp. 130–132*)

40. **(c)** Giving oxygen to a person who is pickwickian will result in respiratory arrest. The hypercarbia that is a feature of the disease dulls the respiratory center and makes it responsive only to hypoxia. (*p. 134*)

41. **(b)** If vitamin A is low, vitamin D usually is, too. (*pp. 134–136*)

42. **(a)** Hypervitaminosis D causes hypotonia, anorexia, irritability, constipation, polyuria, polydipsia, and pallor. (*p. 136*)

43. **(c); 44. (e); 45. (f); 46. (d); 47. (a)** These deficiency diseases are rarely seen in the United States but occur in developing countries. (*pp. 134–145*)

48. **(a); 49. (e); 50. (f); 51. (c)** Pyridoxine deficiency is part of the differential diagnosis of neonatal seizures; pseudoparalysis occurs secondary to painful bone lesions; the "rachitic rosary" is equivalent to enlarged costochondral junctions; the classic triad of pellagra is dematitis, diarrhea, and dementia. (*pp. 134–145*)

52. **(d)** Vitamin D increases calcium mobilization, not reabsorption from bone. (*p. 142*)

53. **(b)** Vitamin E deficiency causes increased platelet adhesiveness. (*p. 146*)

54. **(e); 55. (e); 56. (c); 57. (a)** This infant is not described in the text but was a patient I had seen with a case of severe vitamin K deficiency—hemorrhagic disease of the newborn. The next most likely diagnosis is child abuse; most infants in coma with retinal hemorrhages have been shaken, so skeletal survey is appropriate. The combination of home delivery (no AquaMEPHYTON administered) and the amoxicillin treatment eliminating normal bacterial synthesis of vitamin K led to the tragic demise of an otherwise normal infant. Of all possible preventive measures, the administration of vitamin K at birth would have been most effective.

5

Preventive Pediatrics and Epidemiology

1. (A); 2. (B); 3. (A); 4. (B); 5. (B) Primary prevention implies taking action before an adverse event occurs. Thus, immunization against tetanus and fluoridation are primary actions. Since Pap smears, looking for scoliosis, and measuring lead levels in the blood are all after-the-fact and attempts to prevent further or severe problems, they are examples of secondary prevention. (*pp. 148–154*)

6. (b) Mass screening of children for hypertension has not been shown to be beneficial. The other choices can be most safely and efficiently implemented by the community. (*p. 148*)

7. (a) Encouraging parents to do things that will prevent accidents is nice, but mandatory government controls and/or voluntary manufacturer's actions have been far more effective (*p. 149*)

8. (b) Poisoning primarily affects the 1- to 4-year-old age group. (*p. 149*)

9. (c) Most new parents are not particularly interested in what will happen in the first year, until *after* the baby is born. Focusing on diseases that their as-yet-unborn infant might get is not appropriate. (*p. 150*)

10. (c) I disagree with the text here. The first visit should probably be at 1 week for first mothers, although 2 weeks or occasionally later might be fine for experienced mothers. There is more to "well child" care than immunizations, and anticipatory guidance is important at all ages. (d) is not correct, since in many cases every other year is adequate for the scheduling of health maintenance in the school-aged child. (*p. 150—Tables 5–5 A and B*)

11. (a) is not a true statement. Most pediatricians spend a lot of time in parent education, even if we can't prove it is effective. (*p. 150*)

12. (c) MMR is not recommended until 15 months of age, and smallpox is no longer recommended. Td is used for children over 6 years and for adults. By the time of publication, a form of Hib may be available for use under 1 year of age. (*p. 151—Table 5–5B*)

13. (b) The third and fourth doses are "fillers," except along the Mexican border of the United States, where a third dose is given at 6 months and the fourth and fifth are fillers. OPV is preferred for routine use, but must *not* be used in homes of immuno-compromised children. IPV is given on the same schedule as OPV and is not required for adult contacts of OPV recipients. (*p. 151*)

14. (b); 15. (a); 16. (b); 17. (b) Children with severe chronic sickle cell disease may also benefit from influenza vaccine but should get pneumococcal vaccine to prevent complications of functional asplenia. (*pp. 153–154*)

18. (d) Descriptive epidemiology records prevalence and incidence. Experimental epidemiology measures the effects of a preventive or therapeutic measure. A prospective study could not be done in the case in question. (*pp. 155–156*)

19. (c) Retrospective studies can only provide an estimate of relative risk. (*p. 155*)

20. (c); 21. (a) Observational bias occurs when either the control or the study group is observed more intently. It is important for pediatricians to understand these concepts before initiating or changing practices. (*p. 156*)

22. (b) Diarrhea and malnutrition account for 33 to 50% of mortality. Adequate immunization could reduce the toll of (a)—33%—but systems are not available to deliver them. Not discussed, but a problem for many children, is war, especially in Lebanon, Angola, and other areas. (*pp. 158–159*)

23. (b) Car seats or restraints, not seat belts, are appropriate for infants. (*p. 149*)

24. (c) A tricycle is okay, but most 2- to 4-year-olds do not have the coordination to ride a two-wheeler and should not be riding one. (*p. 149*)

25. (e) is appropriate for a 2- to 4-year-old, but not a school-aged child. (*p. 149*)

(Note: for questions 23–25, see also pp. 216–218)

26. (B); 27. (A); 28. (C); 29. (B); 30. (C); 31. (B); 32. (A); 33. (B); 34. (B); 35. (A); 36. (A); 37. (A); 38. (B); 39. (B); 40. (B) Although these may seem trivial, the reality is that there are contraindications to the use of live viral vaccines in certain populations (e.g., the immunocompromised), so it is better to know what you are administering. When in doubt, read the package insert (*p. 166—Table 5-7*)

6

General Considerations in the Care of the Sick Child

1. **(c)** Some laboratory values vary in the newborn period, but most are similar to adults. The history, developmental considerations, and order of the physical exam to adapt to a child's mood do vary considerably from the adult.

2. **(b)** The abdomen should be auscultated *prior* to palpation and percussion to assess the presence (or absence) of bowel sounds. While not done often, the head should be auscultated to assess the presence of bruits.

3. **(c)** It makes little sense to provide ipecac to the mother of a newborn. When she sees the baby reach for and put objects in his or her mouth, the importance of this piece of anticipatory guidance will be more relevant. Immunizations are not given at all visits (e.g., 2 weeks, 9 months, 3 years) nor is the DDST used after age 5 years. (*p. 173*)

4. **(a)** Pneumonia is most common in this series of 996 febrile infants. The diagnostic value of this data may vary with season and location. (*Table 6–1, p. 174*)

5. **(c)** is correct. TBW is 78% at birth but declines to 60% by 1 year of age (the adult level). (*p. 176*)

6. **(a)** ECF is greater than ICF in fetal life and for the first few months following birth. (*p. 176*)

7. **(b)** Intestinal water is 15% of body weight, plasma water 5%, and gastrointestinal secretions 1 to 3% (fasting state). (*p. 177*)

8. **(d)** GI losses are not considered obligatory. The others are (although if you live in Denver your evaporative losses will be higher than those who live by the sea). (*p. 177*)

9. **(a)** ADH release is stimulated by hemorrhage, leading to decreased urine flow. Osmolality and evaporative water loss do not change with hemorrhage. (*pp. 178–179*)

10. **(c)** ADH is secreted by the supraoptic nuclei, but acts on the renal collecting ducts. (*p. 178*)

11. **(d)** (a), (b), and (c) stimulate ADH release. (*p. 178*)

12. **(d)** Albumin is the only colloid listed and effects water movement. Elevated free fatty acids can cause pseudohyponatremia. (*p. 179*)

13. **(a)** There is little sodium absorption in the stomach. It increases through the the the duodenum and is maximum in the jejunum. (*p. 179*)

14. **(d)** Bile has the highest sodium concentration of transcellular fluid; saliva is highest in potassium. (*p. 182—Table 6–2*)

15. **(a)** The glomerulus filters, but does not reabsorb, sodium (*pp. 180–181*)

16. **(b)** Aldosterone increases blood pressure; it acts on the *distal* tubules. (*p. 181*)

17. **(a)** Skin and muscle are relatively uninvolved in potassium regulation. (*pp. 183–184*)

18. **(e)** Very small increases in total body potassium can lead to hyperkalemia. (*p. 184*)

19. **(d)** Phytate, citrate, and oxalate decrease calcium absorption by complexing the calcium ion. (*p. 185*)

20. **(d)** Malabsorption, hyperparathyroidism, and hypophosphatemia are all associated with hypocalcemia. (*p. 185*)

21. **(b)** Magnesium sulfate is used to treat eclamptic mothers, and newborns can become hypermagnesemic. (*pp. 186, 1348*)

22. **(d)** Bartter syndrome (as well as excessive intake of licorice) causes an alkalosis. (*p. 189*)

23. **(a)** The loss of hydrogen ions in prolonged vomiting leads to a metabolic alkalosis. (*p. 189*)

24. **(b)** The other responses are all associated with hypoventilation and, therefore, a respiratory acidosis. (*p. 190*)

25. **(c)** 100 cal/kg for the first 10 kg, then 50 cal/kg for the next 4 kg. This is the "simplified" method and is acceptable for most cases. It assumes 100 ml of water for 100 cal/kg. (*p. 196, Table 6-7*)

26. **(b)** Since this phase involves ridding the body of excess edema fluid, one need not keep up with the losses. (*p. 197*)

27. **(d)** would be unexpected. With significant dehydration, hemoconcentration occurs. A child with a hematocrit of 28% is significantly anemic. In such a case, one should consider transfusion as an adjunct to fluid rehydration. (*pp. 200–201*)

28. **(d)** Isotonic saline with glucose is best of the choices given and is probably better than normal saline alone when acidosis is present. If you answered (e), you need to reread the whole section. (*p. 201*)

29. **(c)** Patients with gastric distension, uncontrollable vomiting, severe fatigue, stupor, coma, or shock should not receive oral treatment. (*p. 201*)

30. **(b)** is more likely. (e) is possible, and when in doubt repeat lab tests, but such a repeat here would confirm the finding. (*p. 189*)

31. **(c)** is the most important variable. (*p. 235*)

32. **(b)** The treatment of salicylism calls for alkalinization and forced diuresis, since the salicylate is quickly excreted in an alkaline urine. (*pp. 206–207*)

33. **(a)** Premature infants, especially those with respiratory distress, are at greatest risk for neonatal tetany, as are infants of diabetic mothers and those born following a difficult delivery. They usually become symptomatic within 36 hours of birth. (*p. 212*)

34. **(c)** Extensive laboratory evaluation is only indicated after a period of hospitalization in which little weight gain occurs despite adequate caloric intake. In my own experience, many mothers of FTT babies have a past history of being incest victims, although this is not listed in the text. (*pp. 214–215*)

35. **(c)** Infusion of potassium (with the upper limit of 3 mEq/kg/24 hr) will reverse hypokalemia. (*p. 210*)

36. **(e)** The resin used in Kayexalate, 1 gm/kg/24 hr, orally. (*p. 210*)

37. **(f)** Calcium gluconate will reverse the symptoms of hypermagnesemia. (*p. 211*)

38. **(b)** With this extreme level of hypernatremia, dialysis is the best choice. (*p. 210*)

39–48 (*pp. 230–233*)

39. **(B)** The hypertonic fluid draws water into the lungs.

40. **(C)** Seawater by drawing fluid into alveoli; freshwater by causing atelectasis.

41. **(A)** Plasma is diluted with freshwater.

42. **(B)** Seawater is high in chloride.

43. **(C)** Related to the hypoxemia.

44. **(A)**

45. **(A)** Secondary to hypotonicity.

46. **(D)** Such therapy would be harmful in any drowning victim.

47. **(D)** No evidence.

48. **(C)** Initially, few changes may be seen; later, atelectasis, pneumothorax, or shock lung may become apparent.

49. **(a and c)** Impaired myocardial contractility does not occur until later. ADH is stimulated, not inhibited, in burns. (*p. 233*)

50. **(e)** is the only one that can wait. (*p. 234*)

51. **(c)** Respiratory depressants should be avoided. (*p. 234*)

52. **(d)** Calculate using formula on page 235.

53. **(b)** Usually *Pseudomonas* or staphylococcal infection. (*p. 237*)

54. **(c)** And if you can't draw blood, that's a good indication of no venous pressure. Don't try forever. Start fluids by "cut-down" if necessary, and the veins will be more accessible soon.

55. **(c)** (a) is normal, (b) is hypernatremic, and (d) is not compatible with life.

56. **(b)** Boiled skim milk should never be prescribed for diarrhea because of the high association with hypernatremia.

57. **(b)** initially, (a) over the longer term. In a child who is 10% dehydrated, a CVP line is rarely necessary, and the blood pressure is normal.

58. (a) Hypovolemia is first, septic shock second in frequency. With the increase in cardiac surgery, cardiogenic shock is more common. Anaphylaxis and CNS injury are not common. (*pp. 221–222*)

59. (d) Patients with autologous marrow do not reject their own marrow. HLA-identical siblings may still have rejection episodes unless they are identical twins. Older child renal transplant patients (10 to 15 years old) do better than infants. (*pp. 239–245*)

60. (b) Neonates *do* feel pain. Their inability to tell us verbally does not mean it is not present. Opiates are excellent analgesics. The *presence* of parents reduces anxiety (usually) and thus the need for large doses of analgesia. (*p. 250*)

61. (a) The others are pharmacokinetic. (*p. 252*)

62. (a) Individual pharmacokinetics vary too greatly to rely on levels. (*pp. 256–257*)

63. (a) Neomycin is not absorbed by the maternal gut. (*p. 428, Table 9–5*)

64. (e) Ultrasound is less effective when bone or gas is present. (*p. 260*)

65. (d) A CT is approximately 1.0 Rad (over 1 second). A chest film is 0.004. By comparison, a jet pilot absorbs 1 Rad from cosmic rays in 1 year. (*p. 262—Table 6–39*)

66. (b) The MRI is most useful in assessing non-acute head trauma; CT is overused for headache; barium swallows have been replaced by endoscopy; and ultrasound has replaced cholangiography (*p. 261—Table 6–40*)

7

Prenatal Disturbances

1. **(b)** Only about 10% of DNA is represented by genes. (*p. 263*)

2. **(b)** By definition, a polymorphism has no impact on health and disease, and mutations and translocations can occur in both germ and somatic cells. (*p. 265*)

3. **(e)** Delayed mutation has been postulated, but not proved. (*p. 270*)

4. **(b)** 0.5% of newborns have an inborn error of metabolism or sex chromosome abnormality that causes no physical abnormality and can be detected by laboratory test only. (*p. 270*)

5. **(a)** (b) defines a gene locus, (c) a dominant gene, and (d) a recessive gene. (*p. 271*)

6. **(b)**; 7. **(a)**; 8. **(a)**; 9. **(c)**; 10. **(c)**; 11. **(b)**; 12. **(d)**; 13. **(b)**; 14. **(a)**; 15. **(c)**; 16. **(c)**; 17. **(c)** I'm not sure memorizing all of these is necessary, but parents often do ask. If you got any wrong, you would be better off referring to the text before counseling parents. (*pp. 272–273—Table 7–1*)

18. **(c)** The chance of passing the gene is 50%, and the chance of passing the disease is 25%. Consanguinity *doubles* the risk. (*p. 272*).

19. **(b)** Since males determine sex by contributing either an "X" or a "Y" chromosome, a son must receive the Y from his father. Thus, fathers are *never* affected, whereas grandfathers may be affected. (*p. 273*)

20. **(c)** Sex predilection does occur (e.g., pyloric stenosis in males), so (a) is false; (b) is false as well, since identical twins may not be affected at all. (d) is not true either, since the more severe the abnormality, the greater the risk it will also occur in a sibling. (*pp. 273–274*)

21. **(b)** 23 is the haploid number. 46 would be diploid. (*p. 277*)

22. **(c)** Although when there are 69 chromosomes, the cell is both euploid and polyploid. (*p. 279*)

23. **(c)** Aneuploid cells have chromosomal numbers other than multiples of the haploid. (*p. 279*)

24. **(d)** Monosomy results from anaphase lag, nondisjunction increases with age, and pure polyploidy is lethal, not rare. (*p. 279*)

25. **(c)** In reciprocal translocations, all the genetic material is present. (*p. 279*)

26. **(b)** is true, (a) is false. The reason for the observation of increased incidence in younger women is not known. Only 5% of translocations are from carriers, so (c) is false. Congenital heart disease is a feature, usually septal and endocardial cushion defects, and the risk of Down syndrome at age 35 is about one-fourth of 1%. (*pp. 282–284*)

27. **(e)** Probably not of overwhelming importance but interesting in that this is a biochemical marker for Down syndrome. (*p. 284*)

28. **(a)** All trisomies are associated with increased age. 18p is the *only* deletion so associated. As an aside, Klinefelter syndrome is, but Turner syndrome is not. (*pp. 284, 286, 289*)

29. **(a)** (d) is partially true in that these syndromes all have an increased incidence of leukemia, but they are recessive, not dominant. (*p. 291*)

30. **(a)** (b) and (c) are also true statements but not of the Lyon hypothesis. (c) is false, since either maternal or paternal X's may be active (*p. 292*)

31. **(b)** See Answer 28. (*p. 293*)

32. **(a)** This is a minor malformation that needs no work-up. Family history might reveal the same defect in one of the parents. (*p. 295—Table 7–11*)

33. **(b)** This sounds like a congenital infection rather than a chromosomal problem. Isolation precautions are necessary to protect pregnant women from handling the infant. Maternal diabetes leads to large infants.(*p. 299—Table 7–12*)

34. (d) Thalidomide leads to phocomelia, not microcephaly. (*p. 299—Table 7–12*)

35. (e) Tetracycline causes enamel dysplasia when taken in the second and third trimesters. (*p. 299—Table 7–12*)

36. (d) X-rays should be avoided whenever possible, but especially barium enemas, which produce the most radiation. (*p. 300*)

37. (c) Down syndrome is a multiple malformation syndrome. The others are all single defects.(*p. 302*)

38. (d); 39. (b); 40. (c) Fragile-X syndrome is characterized in males by macro-orchidism. Klinefelter's patients have small testes. While fragile-X patients are fertile (in case you answered 40.[d]), they do have a phenotypic pattern mentioned in the literature but not the text. (*p. 295*)

8

Inborn Errors of Metabolism

1. **(b)** Pernicious vomiting is not a sign of glycogen storage disease but is often found in the metabolic acidemias. (*p. 305—Table 8–1*)

2. **(c)** As above, propionic acidemia presents as pernicious vomiting. (*p. 305—Table 8–1*)

3. **(c)** The incidence is 1:14,000, the disease is autosomal recessive, and urine tests are negative at birth. Dietary control is recommended for at least 6 years and probably longer. It is required for pregnant women with PKU. (*pp. 307–310*)

4. **(e)** Most children with PKU have blond hair and blue eyes, but this is not diagnostic. (*p. 307*)

5. **(a)** This form is caused by delayed maturation of *p*-hydroxyphenylpyruvic oxidase. It is autosomal recessive in transmission. (*pp. 310–311*)

6. **(c); 7. (d); 8. (d); 9. (c); 10. (b); 11. (d)** Hartnup disease is a rare disorder of tryptophan metabolism. Alcaptonuria and oculocutaneous albinism are two of the multiple forms of tyrosine disorders. Indicanuria is also tryptophan related and causes blue diaper syndrome. MSUD is a disorder of valine metabolism. Richner-Hanhart syndrome is also known as tyrosenemia type III or oculocutaneous tyrosinemia. (*pp. 310–316*)

12. **(e)** Vitamin B_6 in high doses will lead to improvement in symptoms. (*p. 313*)

13. **(d)** Pyridoxine deficiency is rare, and primary hyperoxaluria is rarer still. Although ethylene glycol ingestion is possible it is more likely that the oxalate crystals have a dietary origin. (*p. 324*)

14. **(e)** Histidase is not part of the urea cycle. (*p. 328, Fig. 8–12*)

15. **(c); 16. (e); 17. (a); 18. (d); 19. (b); 20. (f)** While it is sometimes useful to remember these answers for founds, the likelihood of your being able to do so is only slightly greater than your chance of actually having the opportunity to experience the odors. (*p. 306—Table 8–3*)

21. **(b)** MCAD is the most common. LCAD, SCAD, and MADD are less frequent. **(d)** is a disorder of fatty acid transport. (*p. 336*)

22. **(b)** See Table 8–8 for the list of clinical manifestations of Zellweger syndrome. (*p. 340*)

23. **(b)** Tay Sachs is a GM_2 gangliosidosis Type 1. Type 2 is Sandhoff disease. Type 3 is called juvenile GM_2 gangliosidosis and has later onset. (*pp. 345–347*)

24. **(a)** Fabry disease is also X-linked. (*p. 348*)

25. **(c)** The incidence of Gaucher's disease is most common in Ashkenazi Jews, but the disease has been observed in many other ethnic groups. (*p. 348*)

26. **(a)** Although foam cells are found in the brain, neurologic findings do not cause mortality. (*pp. 349–351*)

27. **(c)** Cholesterol values increase in the newborn period, and are very similar in boys and girls throughout childhood, although HDL drops in males (not females) in the second decade. (*p. 354—Table 8–11*)

28. **(d)** A "prudent diet" is imprudent in children under 2 years. Zealous attempts to restrict fat intake in infancy has led to failure to thrive. (*p. 355*)

29. **(c)** Fruit juices and Kool-Aid contain table sugar (sucrose). Milk has lactose.

30. **(a)** Late-onset disease is found in 70% of black Americans and 10% of Caucasian Americans and does not seem to affect northern Europeans. The symptoms develop gradually and are related to milk and ice cream, not fruit juice. (*p. 983*)

31. **(b)** Lactose is a reducing sugar, but unless it is hydrolyzed it will not react with glucose oxidase.

32. **(c)** Sucrose is nonreducing until hydrolyzed.

33. **(d)** When hydrolyzed to glucose and fructose, both test will be positive.

34. **(b)** The uridyl transferase deficiency is the "classic" form. (*p. 360*)

35. **(a)** Galactitol is thought to be responsible for the cataracts. (*p. 361*)

36. **(a)** This is the only type associated with lactic acidosis. (*pp. 366–377—Table 8–12*)

37. **(d)** All other forms of GSD (including IXa) are autosomal recessive. (*p. 370*)

38. **(d)** Although some enzymes are tissue specific and diagnosis relies on the proper biopsy site, tissue analysis is the only precise diagnostic tool. (*p. 359*)

39. **(C)**; 40. **(C)**; 41. **(B)**; 42. **(D)**; 43. **(A)**; 44. **(D)**; 45. **(B)** Children with Sanfilippo syndrome excrete heparan alone. Scheie and Marateaux-Lamy syndrome children excrete dermantan alone, Hurler and Hunter syndrome urines have both, while keratan sulfate (with or without chondroitin sulfate) is excreted in Morquio syndrome. (*pp. 373–377*)

46. **(d)** Type I glycogen storage disease is associated with gout. (*p. 378*)

47. **(b)** The mechanism for this is unknown but is *not* a result of an inability to feel pain. (*p. 378*)

48. **(c)** This is the highly specific test measuring urinary porphobilinogen in acute intermittent porphyria. (*p. 388*)

49. **(b)** Blacks have 20 to 30% of the incidence of Type I diabetes mellitus seen in Caucasians. The sex ratio is equal, onset is usually autumn or winter, and the prevalence is approximately 2/1000 in school-aged children with 16 new cases/100,000 children. (*p. 391*)

50. **(c)** The precise etiology is not clear, but an autoimmune reaction triggered by a viral infection in a "susceptible" host seems best to tie most of the theories together. There is no relationship to diet, exercise, or maturity-onset diabetes. Although there is a link to certain HLA types, autosomal recessive inheritance is not proved. (*pp. 392–393*)

51. **(b)**, **(c)**, **(e)** There is some insulin present, and cholesterol is elevated. (*p. 394*)

52. **(c)**, **(d)**, **(e)** Most children present with polyuria, polydipsia, polyphagia, and weight loss. 75% of children have partial remission. (*pp. 394–395*)

53. **(a)**, **(b)** The diagnosis of IDDM is dependent on unexplained (i.e., no other etiology such as trauma) hyperglycemia and glycosuria. Ketoacidosis is not necessary for diagnosis. (*p. 395*)

54. **(a)**, **(b)**, **(d)** Maintenance of continuous normoglycemia is not feasible and, to date, neither is prevention of microvascular disease. (*pp. 397–404*)

55. **(a)**, **(b)** Regular insulin preparations have an onset at ½ hour, peaking at 2 to 4 hours. Ultralente and P21 have delayed onset (4 to 8 hours) and peak at 14 to 20 hours. (*p. 399—Table 8–21*)

56. **(c)** Onset is rapid, with pallor, sweating, and tachycardia. They should be acutely aborted with carbohydrate (candy, non-diet sodas) and exercise and/or diminished insulin. (*p. 403*)

57. **(a)**, **(b)**, **(d)** Hypoglycemia alternates with hyperglycemia; dwarfism has not been related. (*p. 404*)

58. **(b)**, **(c)** Adrenal insufficiency occurs in the second decade if it is to happen. (*p. 407*)

59. **All** are appropriate.

60. **(d)** A semicomatose patient should be brought directly to the hospital.

61. **(a)**, **(c)**, **(d)**, **(e)** Subcutaneous insulin is not useful in ketoacidotic patients.

62. **(d)**; 63. **(b)**; 64. **(b)**; 65. **(c)**; 66. **(b)**; 67. **(c)**; 68. **(d)** There may be some local variations in approach, but the general principles of management of ketoacidosis apply here. (*pp. 395–402*)

69. **(a)**, **(b)** Leucine sensitivity is probably nesidioblastosis. The ACD blood effect occurs 2 to 3 hours after transfusion. (*p. 413*)

70. **(b)**, **(c)**, **(e)** Onset is usually 18 months to 5 years. A link to panhypopituitarism is not known. (*p. 414*)

9
The Fetus and the Neonatal Infant

1. (c) The NMRs for white and black infants are approximately double the figures given, which are the postneonatal mortality rates. (*p. 421*)

2. (c) Risk assessment is important for appropriate prenatal care. (*p. 429*)

3. (b) The highest are (a) and (d). (*p. 429*)

4. (c) The L/S ratio will estimate maturity. Ultrasound can estimate size, but has its limitations—it told us that our fourth was "about 36 week size." Seven weeks later he was born at term and 9 lbs. 4 oz. Few people are "average." (*p. 436*)

5. (d) A low L/S ratio is only predictive of hyaline membrane disease 75 to 80% of the time. Neither maternal nor fetal blood contamination will affect the test, although meconium will. Maternal diabetes and hydrops will decelerate pulmonary maturation (and thus lower the ratio). (*p. 436*)

6. (a) Renal hypoplasia is associated with oligohydramnios, and midforceps deliveries are associated with traumatic injury, not anoxia. (*pp. 429–431*)

7. (c) Wormian bones are associated with osteogenesis imperfecta, cleidocranial dysostosis, congenital hypothyroidism, and occasionally Down syndrome. (*pp. 423–425*)

8. (c) One off for color. (*p. 427—Table 9–3*)

9. (a) Daily hexachlorophene bathing has been associated with neurotoxicity. A single bath will suffice if there is a staph aureus epidemic. (*p. 427*)

10. (c), (d) Propranol and propylthiouracil are probably safe, as is methadone, although it could sedate the newborn. (*p. 428—Table 9–5*)

11. (d) (a) is premature, (b) is small for gestational age, (c) is premature and large for gestational age, and (e) is large for gestational age. (*p. 440*)

12. (c) Twins of the same sex may be either monozygotic or dizygotic. Perinatal mortality is significantly (fourfold) higher. (*pp. 439–440*)

13. (a) Prematurity is a condition, not a cause of death. (*p. 443*)

14. (c) Blacks have nearly double the rate of VLBW infants. These VLBW infants account for 50% of the neonatal deaths (not the overwhelming majority) and although they can be SGA, prematurity is the usual condition. (*p. 442*)

15. (b) AGA infants are less likely to become hypoglycemic than either SGA infants or infants of diabetic mothers. (*p. 444—Fig. 9–11*)

16. (d) Handwashing, not incubators, controls infection. (*p. 445*)

17. (a) Gastrostomy is associated with high morbidity and mortality rates. (*pp. 446–447*)

18. (b) All of the choices listed are possible complications of intravenous hyperalimentation, but hyperglycemia will lead to an osmotic diuresis, dehydration, and azotemia. (*pp. 447–448*)

19. (a) This is probably an editorial opinion rather than "hard data," but it is also probably true. (*p. 448*)

20. (e) Hemorrhage leads to pallor, not cyanosis; parenthetically, cyanosis may occur in a severely anemic infant. (*p. 452*)

21. (a) Fever is most often the result of overheating or overdressing. Although infection can lead to a fever, the usual symptoms are hypothermia and difficulty in maintaining a normal body temperature. (*p. 453*)

22. (a) See Answer 21.

23. (e) If the vomiting and diarrhea were caused by disease, the infant would not look well and would probably be dehydrated with little urine output. (*p. 453*)

24. **(e)** The definition of a cephalohematoma requires that it be confined to a bone. Caput succedaneum, which is primarily edema fluid, will cross suture lines. (*p. 454*)

25–27. **(b), (a), (d)** Erb-Duchenne is more common than Klumpke's paralysis. Both involve the brachial plexus, but the upper plexus is more often injured. Facial paralysis is, obviously, cranial nerve VII related (the "Finn" On Old Olympus' Topmost Top in the anatomy mnemonic). (*pp. 456–457*)

28. **(a)** Not only are clavicular fractures most common, but they are often unnoticed until a large callus is felt by the parent at one week of age. All of the injuries in Questions 25 through 28 are related to difficult deliveries secondary to abnormal presentations or obstetric trauma. (*p. 457*)

29. **(b)** Choanal atresia or any upper airway obstruction will lead to the symptoms described. (*p. 459*)

30. **(e)** is the only correct answer. (*p. 462*)

31. **(e)** is false. It was true in the old days. (*pp. 463–464*)

32. **(b)** CPAP should be tried if 70% oxygen is unsuccessful in reversing hypoxemia. If CPAP fails, assisted ventilation may be necessary. See Question 33. (*p. 464*)

33. **(c)** Assuming CPAP has failed. See Question 32. (*p. 465*)

34. **(d)** Pulmonary artery stenosis is a congenital problem. (*pp. 466–468*)

35. **(c)** Unless the PFC is accompanied by a diaphragmatic hernia. (*p. 471*)

36. **(d)** The other name for this is type II respiratory distress syndrome. (*p. 469*)

37. **(d)** The obstruction in (a) and (b) prohibits bilious vomiting, and the intact pylorus in (c) makes it unlikely. Bilious vomiting is a four-star emergency. (*p. 474*)

38. **(b)** Meconium plugs, ileus and *peritonitis* may be indicative of cystic fibrosis. (*p. 475*)

39. **(b)** Rotavirus infection, along with *Clostridium difficile, C. perfringens* and *Escherichia coli*, have been associated with some cases, but are not solely etiologic. (*p. 476*)

40. **(b)** The other three choices are pathologic, not physiologic. (*pp. 477–478*)

41. **(d)** No treatment is necessary assuming normal growth and development. If the mother tires of people stopping her in the supermarket commenting on how yellow her baby looks, a short time off the breast will resolve this problem. (*pp. 478–479*)

42. **(e)** The hypothyroid baby is lethargic, but not opisthotonic, and has a low cry. (*p. 492*)

43. **(b)** (c) occurs simultaneously, but when conjugated hyperbilirubinemia is present without phototherapy, the "bronze" color is not present. (*p. 481*)

44. **(c)** In (a) and (b), the liver will probably begin conjugating any time. (d) is probably prolonged hyperbilirubinemia of breast feeding and need not be treated. (*pp. 484–485*)

45. **(b)** Congenital spherocytosis presents later. (*pp. 481–482*)

46. **(b)** The D antigen is the culprit in most Rh disease. The others are minor. (*p. 482*)

47. **(a)** (c) is false because ABO sensitization protects against the effects of Rh. Administration of human anti-D globulin will prevent the disease. (*pp. 483–485*)

48. **(c)** Jaundice occurs later. (*p. 483*)

49. **(a)** In this emergency situation, Rh-negative blood crossmatched to the mother will do. Later, infant type-specific blood should be used. (*p. 485*)

50. **(b)** Only IgG antibody crosses the placenta. The incompatibility is more common, although severe hemolytic disease is less common than in Rh disease. (*p. 486*)

51. **(a)** These are the vitamin K-dependent factors and return to normal at 7 to 10 days. (*p. 486*)

52. **(c)** Beware of home-delivered babies who may not get vitamin K. (*p. 487*)

53. **(b)** Fetal Hb is alkali resistant. (*p. 487*)

54. **(b)** This is a rarely seen umbilical polyp. The discharge is urine-like. (*p. 489*)

55. **(a)** Surgery is unnecessary, strapping is ineffective, and strangulation never occurs. (*p. 489*)

56. **(e)** Magnesium sulfate treatments of eclamptic mothers yields hypermagnesemia in babies. (*p. 490*)

57. **(d)** The tremors are possible with all the choices, but the diarrhea and nasal stuffiness distinguish the syndrome. (*pp. 490–491*)

58. **(d)** Phenobarbital is the treatment of choice for heroin withdrawal. (*p. 491*)

59. **(d)** The incidence of hyaline membrane disease is higher in infants of diabetic mothers. (*pp. 492–493*)

60. **(e)** Hypoparathyroidism predisposes to hypocalcemia. (*pp. 493–494*)

61. **(b)** The incidence of amnionitis after premature rupture of membranes goes up *after* 24 hours, maternal antibody is protective, and urinary tract infections are more common than sepsis, so (a), (c), and (d) are false. (*pp. 495–496*)

62. **(b)** *Chlamydia* infections are acquired postnatally. (*pp. 498, 505*)

63. **(a)** Hepatitis B is usually symptomatic in adults. CMV, HSV-2 and rubella are generally asymptomatic. (*pp. 505, 517, 519, 521*)

64. **(c)** Usually the maternal and newborn samples have approximately the same titer, and the 3-month serum will fall if there is no infection and stay elevated or rise if there is infection. *All three must be analyzed at the same time.* (*p. 498*)

65. **(d)** These measures will find *Pseudomonas*. (*pp. 500–501*)

66. **(c)** Staph, strep, and *Haemophilus* strike older infants and children; *Pseudomonas* and *Klebsiella* are less common. (*p. 502*)

67. **(a)** is a minimum with smaller quantities of broth and will probably grow organisms if sepsis is present, but (d) is optimal. (*p. 503*)

68. **(b)** is acceptable. Sulfa drugs are unacceptable in newborns, so (a) is never true. (d) might apply if a staph epidemic is in progress. Erythromycin is an orally administered drug and therefore not acceptable for the treatment of sepsis. (*p. 502, Table 9–31*)

69. **(d)** Prophylactic antibiotics are an answer. Maternal immunization may be in the future. (*p. 512*)

70. **(c)** *Staphylococcus aureus* is the most common agent in osteomyelitis at any age. (*p. 692*)

71. **(a)** After the newborn period, female UTI predominates. (*p. 509*)

72. **(a)** Chemical is early (less than 24 hrs of age), infectious late. (*p. 504*)

73. **(b)** Only one-third of infections are caused by these organisms in neonates. *Escherichia coli, Klebsiella pneumoniae, Pseudomonas aeruginosa, Staphylococcus aureus*, and group B *Streptococcus* are the usual etiologic agents. (*p. 507*)

74. **(A); 75. (C); 76. (D); 77. (A); 78. (B); 79. (A)** The mortality is higher in early-onset disease (60 to 90%), but the rate (15 to 40%) for late onset is still extremely high. (*pp. 509–513*)

80. **(d)** Nosocomial transmission of CMV in the nursery is rare. (*p. 514*)

81. **(b)** These infants are at risk if breast fed, but hepatitis B has not been shown to be teratogenic. If the infant becomes a carrier, the antigen will never clear, so HB_SIG is the right choice. (*p. 506*)

82. **(a)** Onset is later than 12 to 24 hours, the skin is almost always involved, and Ara-A is beneficial. (*p. 518*)

83. **(c)** Polioviruses now rarely cause disease, although attenuated vaccine virus is often grown in viral cultures. Enteroviruses do not cause congenital infection. They are common in summer as encephalitis, not meningitis. (*p. 516*)

84. **(b)** The worst time is 0 to 4 days. (*p. 522*)

85. **(b)** Echovirus is an enterovirus. See Answer 83

86–94. The problem presented in these questions is not a hypothetical one. It occurs daily and, although outcomes vary, the major thing to be learned from this case is that the uterus is the best transport incubator, and high-risk deliveries and newborn care need to be done with appropriate staff in the appropriate center.

86. **(a)** and **(b)** are really unacceptable answers, as you will see in Answer 88. (c) is OK, but **(d)** is definitely the best.

87. **(a)–(f), (j),** and **(k)** are important immediately in the management of ill prema-

tures. (g) and (h) are helpful later; (i) probably is unnecessary.

88. In this situation, with a shocky, cold, hypoxic infant, there is little that can be done in an unequipped rural (or urban, for that matter) hospital. (a) and (d) are available to you but only prolong the inevitable. No umbilical catheter is found in this hospital, and the transport team informs you that all ground and air transportation is unavailable because of the storm. Within 2 hours the infant has cardiorespiratory arrest and expires while your inexperienced x-ray technician attempts a chest film.

89. (a) is probably as unacceptable as it was in Answer 86. Even if you are a pediatrician your Level I hospital can only stabilize infants. This one is potentially a disaster, and with the storm coming, it would be best to get either (b) or (c). It just so happens, that in the interest of brevity, we arranged for (b) and (c) to wind up at Level II through Question 90.

91. (a) is a must. You cannot be admitted to any hospital that is accredited in the United States and not get (b). (c) is not available and is probably unnecessary; (d) is indicated to confirm the shake test and shows a 1.3:1 ratio. (e) is unnecessary; (f) is done, as is (g).

92. (a)–(d), (g), and (h) are needed immediately. (e) and (f) can wait.

93. (a) is the proper approach. The infant is too ill for a complete septic work-up, although blood cultures should be done. If you chose (c) you have failed to recognize shock, and the infant will not respond to treatment well. (d) is premature.

94. (a) is correct. (b) is possible, but the reason for inappropriate ADH would be obscure. (c) through (g) are unlikely with the information given.

10

Special Health Problems During Adolescence

1. **(a)** Violence—including accidents, homicides, and suicides—accounts for 70% of all adolescent deaths. Neoplasms account for 7% and infectious diseases and congenital anomalies account for another 7%. While sexually transmitted diseases are very common, they are not often associated with mortality. (*p. 525*)

2. **(e)** automobiles, alcohol, and adolescence has never mixed. All of the statements are true except the last; lowering of the drinking age to 18 years has been associated with a 5% increase in fatal automotive accidents. A drinking age of 21 would be a significant preventive measure. (*p. 525*)

3. **(b)** Acting-out behavior is a hallmark of masked depression. Substance abuse, school truancy, multiple accidents, running away from home, and promiscuity are all symptoms, as are somatic symptoms. (*p. 526*)

4. **(a)** Even though more boys than girls hang, shoot, or slash themselves and use more violent methods, the ingestion route is the most common. (*p. 526*)

5. **(c)** Alcohol is the most widely abused substance. (*p. 527*)

6. **(a)** The effect of estrogen is to decrease metabolism and therefore increase the likelihood of intoxication. (*p. 528, Table 10–2*)

7. **(e)** withdrawal begins within 8 hours and lasts 24 to 36 hours. (*p. 529*)

8. **(d)** the latex fixation test is falsely *positive*. (*p. 529*)

9. **(c); 10. (a); 11. (b); 12. (d); 13. (c); 14. (b)** Marijuana (active component is tetrahydrocannabinol) is also known as pot, hash, grass, or weed. Phencyclidine is the active ingredient of PCP, also known as sternyl, angel dust, hog, peace pill, and sheets. Toluene is the active ingredient of airplane glue and jimsonweed is also known as locoweed, devil's weed, and stinkweed. (*pp. 529–531*)

15. **(c)** Spermatogenesis is also decreased with the use of marijuana 4 times a week for 6 months. (*p. 531*)

16. **(c)** This type of physiologic observation is only recently being appreciated. (*p. 532*)

17. **(b); 18. (a); 19. (b); 20. (a); 21. (c); 22. (c); 23. (b); 24. (a); 25. (d)** Strikingly absent from this discussion in the textbook is any mention of sexual abuse as an etiology and/or associated event in eating disorders in adolescents. (*pp. 533–534*)

26. **(c)** Access to abortion is the primary explanation for the decreased pregnancy rate. In the mid-1980s, the data may show that fear of AIDS will be an important factor. (*p. 534*)

27. **(a)** Gonorrhea is the most reported. (*pp. 536, 717*)

28. **(f); 29. (a); 30. (e); 31. (b); 32. (d)** The dosages are given in the text. It should be remembered that sexually transmitted diseases are not often found in pure form, and multiple therapy is needed. (*pp. 536–537*)

33. **(c)** 60% of girls have menarche at SMR 4, 10% at SMR 2 and SMR 5, and 20% at SMR 3. (*p. 537*)

34. **(c)** The diagnosis will be made by examination revealing a bulging hymen (*p. 538*)

35. **(d)** Enovid therapy is used to stop bleeding. All the other choices are etiologies for menometrorrhagia. (*p. 538*)

36. **(a)** Fibroadenomas (and benign cysts—not a choice here) are most common. Carcinoma is rare, and thus mammography is not indicated. (*p. 540*)

37. **(b)** Gonococcal arthritis is more common in adolescents, but nongonococcal infections (e.g., hemophilus influenza B) are more common in younger children. (*p. 540*)

38. **(d)** Because of the resurgence of measles and rubella among adolescents and young

adults, an MMR reimmunization is now recommended. It is best done in early adolescence. If done later, action should be taken to avoid use of MMR in a pregnant adolescent. Read the package insert with the vaccine. (*p. 540*)

39. (b) Unless emancipated, an adolescent may not donate organs or blood without con-

sent. As of this writing (January, 1992), the Supreme Court has not ruled on question (d), although it has upheld an adolescent's right to privacy. (*p. 541*)

40. (a) Urinalysis (and culture) are useful in females only as a screening method. The rest are important for both genders. (*p. 541*)

11

Immunity, Allergy, and Related Diseases

1. **(a)** Elaboration of immunoglubulins is a B cell function. (*p. 545—Table 11–1*)

2. **(e); 3. (d); 4. (a); 5. (c); 6. (b); 7. (c); 8. (a)** Each of the these immunoglobulins has a different molecular weight and biologic properties, some of which are indicated in the answers to these questions. See Table 11–5 as well as the text. (*pp. 547–548*)

9. **(b)** A negative test. (a) tells you nothing; the presence of large lymphocytes is associated with T-cell deficiency; a retrosternal radiolucency is likely a normal thymus; and one would not expect diminished in vitro PHA response in the normal situation. (*pp. 548–549*)

10. **(a)** Never give live virus vaccines to individuals you suspect have an immune deficiency disease. (*p. 550*)

11. **(d)** Bruton disease does not present with thrombocytopenia. (*p. 555*)

12. **(a); 13 (c); 14. (c); 15. (b); 16. (a); 17. (a); 18. (c)** (*pp. 551–555*)

19. **(b)** The androgen is synthetic (danazol) and is for use in adults only. (*p. 562*)

20. **(c)** In chronic granulomatous disease there is defective oxidative metabolism and production of reactive oxygen radicals; in Chédiak-Higashi syndrome degranulation is abnormal. (*pp. 566–568*)

21. **(e)** Job syndrome is also known as hyperimmunoglobulin E recurrent infection syndrome. (*p. 569*)

22. **(b)** Absolute eosinophilia is a characteristic. (*pp. 570–571*)

23. **(b)** RAST is more convenient than skin testing, but not as sensitive. (*pp. 576–577*)

24. **(c)** Antimicrobial agents have little use except in primary or secondary bacterial infection. (*p. 578*)

25. **(a)** Isoproterenol is not oral, so (b) is incorrect; only theophylline is effective for asthma, so eliminate (c); there is no evidence that antihistamines are deleterious, and cromolyn is for prophylaxis, *not* treatment, of acute attacks. (*pp. 579–582*)

26. **(d)** The every-other-day (AM) regimen minimizes the side effects of steroids. (*p. 584*)

27. **(c)** There are no FDA standards of potency—a real problem. (*pp. 584–585*)

28. **(c)** Allergic rhinitis is followed by asthma in only 3 to 10% of cases; ragweed allergy is rarely seen in children before 4 to 5 years; nasal sympathetomimetics are only effective for a few days—then a rebound effect occurs. Nasal corticosteroids are very effective. (*pp. 586–587*)

29. **(c)** Emotional factors can precipitate an attack but are not primary etiologic and pathophysiologic factors. (*pp. 587–590*)

30. **(b)** Mist tents are useless. They do not deliver water to the lower airway, are irritating to many children, and hide the patient, who needs to be seen. (*pp. 592–594*)

31. **(d)** Intermittent inhaled steroids may be needed in moderate asthma. Alternate-day steroids are reserved for severe asthmatics. (*p. 594*)

32. **(d)** Topical antibiotics may sensitize irritated skin. (*p. 599*)

33. **(e)** Psychogenic factors, if they are present, are secondary. (*p. 600*)

34. **(d)** These entities are common in adults, rare in children. (*p. 601*)

35–41. This problem relates a typical presentation for a child with asthma. If the child had been 6 months old instead of 16, bronchiolitis might have been more likely. Nevertheless, in handling this problem, **(a)** is the proper choice for Question 35. You nearly always need more history.

36. All the historical questions asked are appropriate *except* (h). The differential diagnosis includes bacterial or viral pneumonia, bronchiolitis, foreign body aspiration, and asthma. Cysts and aberrant bronchial rings are unlikely to present so late and so suddenly.

37. (c) In Question 37, as in Question 30, reassurance is not the answer; neither are antibiotics at home nor rapid hospitalization before lab data are obtained.

38. Of all the lab data available, (a), (b), (f), (i), (m), and possibly (n) are mandatory. The rest are plus-minus, except for the lumbar puncture for CSF culture (k), which is just not indicated.

39. The lab results lead you toward asthma and mild hypoxia, good hydration, and no sign of bacterial disease or foreign body aspiration. Time now for (b), a treatment trial (probably not in the hospital, although that will vary).

40. The appropriate sequence is (d)-(b)-(c) or (d)-(e)-(c), either of which clear the wheezing, and the tachypnea and the hypoxia disappear. Oral theophylline will keep the attack under control. Should the initial therapy have failed, then (a) and (f) would have followed. (g) has no place here at all.

41. (d) Obvious by now.

42. (b) Glomerulonephritis is common in rabbits, rare in children. (*pp. 602–603*)

43. (a) 95% of patients with ankylosing spondylitis have HLA B27 in contrast to only 6% of North Americans. Pauciarticular type II is also associated, not type I. (*p. 612*)

44. (c) Aspirin remains the safest and most satisfactory therapy for JRA and should be tried first. (*pp. 618—621*)

45. (d) Renal disease is more common in adults. (*pp. 624–627*)

46. (c) The purpura on the lower extremities gives this away. Meningococcemia is generalized. (*pp. 628–629*)

47. (d) The etiology of Kawasaki disease remains a mystery. Treatment is symptomatic and recovery is usually complete, although 1 to 2% of children die of a coronary vasculitis. (*p. 629*)

48. (d) Controlled studies have shown gamma globulin, intravenously, to reduce the incidence of coronary vasculitis. (*p. 630*)

49. (e) Salicylates are effective for erythema nodosum, antibiotics for Lyme disease. Steroids are not effective for dermatomyositis or scleroderma. (*pp. 633–637*)

50–54. The five major criteria are (b), (d), (e), (g), and (h). (*p. 642—Table 11–40*)

55. (e) No vaccine is yet available. (*pp. 640–641*)

12

Infectious Diseases

1. **(b)** Most children with neoplasia do not have fever alone. Acetaminophen is symptomatic and is not an effective treatment. (*p. 652*)

2. **(b); 3. (d); 4 (a); 5. (c)** The blood agar and Thayer-Martin agar can be routinely plated in office settings. The HI test and Giemsa stains are laboratory procedures and usually done in office settings. (*pp. 658–660*)

6. **(a)** *Yersinia* is invasive, not toxigenic. (*pp. 662–663*)

7. **(d)** Mumps virus used to be the leading cause of aseptic meningitis in the United States in the 1960s. With routine immunization, it now accounts for only 2% of cases. (*p. 665*)

8. **(d)** *H. influenzae* type B is most common. (*p. 683*)

9. **(c); 10. (a); 11. (a); 12. (b); 13. (d); 14. (b).** Limping can occur in either disease. In children with sickle cell disease, salmonella and *S. pneumoniae* are common pathogens (although *Staphyloccus* is still #1). In septic arthritis in a 2-year-old, *H. influenzae* would be most likely. Treatment is 2 to 3 weeks for septic arthritis, 4 to 6 weeks for osteomyelitis. (*pp. 691–698*)

15. **(b)** Infants rarely get pharyngitis but do get nasal discharge and fever. Infection predominates in cold weather, and serious sequelae are rare. Actual immunity status of carriers is controversial. (*p. 700*)

16. **(e)** Bullous pyoderma is caused by staphylococci. (*p. 700–703*)

17. **(c)** An increase in the ASO titer does indicate prior streptococcal infection, but the throat (or nose) culture is quicker, less expensive, and diagnostic. (*p. 701*)

18. **(d)** Tetracycline and sulfonamides are unacceptable for treatment. (*p. 702*)

19. **(a)** Staph does a lot of things, but it doesn't cause tonsillopharyngitis. (*pp. 704–705*)

20. **(a)** is simple and effective and is the correct answer. (*p. 705*)

21. **(b)** Incidence is highest in 2-year-olds, epidemics are sporadic, infection often follows viral infection, and the vaccine works best in children 2 years of age or older. (*pp. 709–711*)

22. **(a)** It was previously said that if you just say the word "penicillin," the pneumococci will die. That is no longer true. Resistance occurs in 2 to 15% of strains. (*p. 711*)

23. **(d)** Polysaccharide vaccines are not immunogenic in infants. (*pp. 711–713*)

24. **(a)** Meningitis is not a bad sign. It indicates ability to respond to the septicemia. (*p. 716*)

25. **(b)** Pen V has only 10 to 25% the efficacy of Pen G. (*p. 716*)

26. **(c)** Gram stain is presumptive only in men; women have other flora that can confuse. (*pp. 716–720*)

27. **(b)** One of the first triumphs of modern preventive medicine. (*pp. 721–724*)

28. **(a)** is false, since it is the toxin that invades. The rest are all true. (*pp. 721–724*)

29. **(d)** One needs *all* the therapeutic stoppers for diptheria. (*pp. 723–724*)

30. **(a)** is true. I know of no controlled studies to prove pertussis immune globulin's effectiveness in treatment. (*p. 726*)

31. **(c)** Only some of the strains have blood and leukocytes. (*pp. 727–729*)

32. **(c)** Salmonellae are inactivated at pH 2. Those with gastrectomies are, therefore, susceptible. (*p. 730*)

33. **(b)** Improving sanitation and housing is the most effective preventive measure in endemic areas. (*pp. 731–734*)

34. **(a)** Ampicillin is the antibiotic of choice for susceptible strains, not neomycin. Man is the reservoir, especially in institutions.

Bactermia is common in *Salmonella*, not *Shigella*. (*pp. 734–736*)

35. (c) The lungs of children with cystic fibrosis are colonized by *Pseudomonas*, but septicemia is rare. (*pp. 738–740*)

36. (c); 37. (d); 38. (a); 39. (b) Knowing vectors and reservoir animals is especially important for those who will practice in rural areas; maybe the only place to earn a living in the 1900s. (*pp. 741–745*)

40. (d) Meningitis is not one of the forms of tuleremia. (*pp. 744–745*)

41. (c) Nonroutine antibiotics for nonroutine infections. (*pp. 741–745*)

42. (b) The presence of early- and late-onset forms of the disease in newborns is most like group B streptococcal infection in newborns. (*p. 746*)

43. (e) Meningitis is secondary to cutaneous anthrax, rarely following the pulmonary form. Hepatic anthrax has not been reported. Take my word for this as Anthrax was dropped from this edition.

44. (c) The case fatality rate hasn't changed much, and tetanospasmin is the endotoxin. Antitoxin does not reverse the effects, and the exotoxin is not immunogenic, so the toxoid should be given to those recovering. (*pp. 747–749*)

45. (e) The others are all indicated in this case, which may be the standard high-risk wound. (*pp. 748–749*)

46. (a) Boiling will inactivate the toxin, not the spores, the inactivation of which requires a pressure cooker at 115.5° C. Antibiotics are a must, vaccine is not available, and newborns do better than adults. (*pp. 752–754*)

47. (c) There must be *no* oxygen for anaerobes to grow well. (*p. 750*)

48. (a) *Bacteroides fragilis* is resistant to penicillin, ampicillin, and cephalosporin. (*p. 756*)

49. (c); 50. (b); 51. (a); 52. (c and d); 53. (e); 54. (a) Each of these opportunistic infections occurs where the normal host defenses are compromised and otherwise "normal flora" become pathogens. (*p. 670, Table 12–14*)

55. (b) Penicillin prophylaxis after the bite is treated locally will prevent this. (*p. 1795*)

56. (c) *Campylobacter* also causes bacteremia. (*p. 757*)

57. (a) Legionnaires' disease with pneumonia predominating. (*p. 760*)

58. (a) A variant of legionnaires', Pontiac fever. (*p. 759*)

59. (d) Sulfur granules are pathognomonic. (*p. 762*)

60. (b) is true. BCG should not be used routinely when less than 10% of the population is tuberculin positive. Children swallow their sputum. Chemotherapy is effective in treatment, not prevention. Miliary TB occurs mostly commonly in infants. (*pp. 763–771*)

61. (b) Triple therapy as outline is the way to go, although the streptomycin may not be needed for very long. (*pp. 766–767*)

62. (d) It is not seen much any more, but the description is classical for congenital syphilis. (*p. 777*)

63. (e) Weil disease is caused by *Leptospira*. (*p. 782*)

64. (d) *Mycoplasma pneumoniae* is a well-known cause of pneumonia. When conjunctivitis is present, *Chlamydia* should be considered. *Mycobacterium tuberculosis* is obvious, and *Rickettsia* (Q fever, Rocky Mountain spotted fever) is yet another cause of pneumonia. *Plasmodium* is not. (*pp. 786–790*)

65. (b) Peak contagiousness occurs just *before* onset of rash. (*pp. 791–793*)

66. (b) is correct. (c) is mumps, (d) is roseola, and (e) is measles. (*p. 794*)

67. (b) is correct. The description sounds like roseola (*p. 796*), *not* erythema infectiosum as in (d), but roseola is not a choice here. (a) is incorrect because the rash in roseola appears *after* the fever falls (usually day 3 to 4). Rubella prodome is usually mild (*p. 794*), so (c) is untrue, and scarlet fever is most often seen in school-aged children.

68. (c) Most neonatal herpes is caused by type 2 herpes. Smallpox immunization does nothing for stomatitis and is hazardous.

Hyperimmune globulin is not available, and adenovirus causes epidemic keratoconjunctivitis. (*pp. 797–800*)

69. (b) Crusts are infectious in smallpox. Lesions of varicella and herpes are indistinguishable. Although the varicella vaccine is not yet approved for routine use, 21G is proven and can be used in special cases. (*pp. 800–803*)

70. (c) Hepatitis A and B are also part of the differential diagnosis is acquired infection. (*pp. 803–805*)

71. (e) Corticosteroids are used for severe tonsillar hypertrophy and significant illness only. (*pp. 805–808*)

72. (c) Infertility is uncommon, although the fear of it is great. The mumps skin test is no longer available, as it was useless. (*pp. 808–810*)

73. (b) Reye syndrome occurs most commonly after influenza B and an association with aspirin has recently been drawn. (*p. 812*)

74. (e) Parainfluenza 4 infection is generally asymptomatic. (*p. 813*)

75. (b) Probably adenovirus 11 or 21. (*p. 816*)

76. (a) RSV causes bronchiolitis; the older the better; transplacental antibody is not protective (hence severe disease in early infancy), and the inactivated vaccine was not only ineffective, but hazardous. (*pp. 814–816*)

77. (b) Hepatitis B is transmitted orally as well as parenterally. Although not referred to in the textbook, it was the classic work of another Krugman that sorted out hepatitis A and B and led to the prophylactic vaccine. (*pp. 818–822*)

78. (e) Poliovirus, coxsackievirus, and echovirus are enteroviruses—a subgroup of picornavirus. (*p. 823*)

79. Of the choices given, **(b)** is the best. New York City is not an area of high rabies incidence. (*p. 834*)

80. (c) This reference is not mentioned in the text. Take my word for the obvious answer.

81. (c) (*p. 860*); **82. (a)** (*p. 849*); **83. (d)** (*p. 859*); **84. (b)** (*p. 860*); **85. (e)** (*p. 860*); **86. (a)** (*p. 852*); **87. (e)** (*p. 858*) Asking for

vectors may seem like nitpicking (!), but these vectors have changed the course of history (see Zinsser's *Rats, Lice and History*).

88. (a) Atypical myobacteria are not fungi. (*pp. 772–774*)

89. (e) No vaccine is available for coccidioidomycosis. (*pp. 870–872*)

90. (a) through (i) are all relevant.

91. (a), (b), (d), (h), (i), (j), (m), (n), (p), and (q) are appropriate for a start. If those are negative, the others can be pursued. The trip to central Missouri is the tip-off to histoplasmosis, since it is endemic in that area.

92. (e) No treatment is needed. The disease is self-limited in older children.

93. (d) Anemia is seen in chronic hookworm infestation. Löeffler-like syndromes and intussusception occur with heavy infestations of *Ascaris*. (*p. 896*)

94. (c) Visceral larva migrans (toxocariasis) causes extraordinarily high eosinophil counts in this form but not in ocular infection. The syndrome of tropical pulmonary eosinophilia (not a choice here) is also part of the differential diagnosis and is caused by microfilariae. (*p. 900*)

95. (c) Echinococcus eggs are ingested. (*p. 907*)

96. (c) To alleviate tick paralysis, one need only remove the tick. Those sensitive to bees should undergo hyposensitization, as there is no antivenin. (*p. 919*)

97. (a) Paragonimiasis is caused by lung fluke (trematode). (*p. 905*)

98. (d) Toxoplasmosis is a common cause of prematurity, blindness (from chorioretinitis), and mental retardation, but *not* cerebral palsy. Most maternal infections are asymptomatic, and any prior exposure will confer passively transferable immunity to subsequent fetuses. (*pp. 883–892*)

99. (b) *Giardia* is now a common etiologic agent out of the Rocky Mountains as well. Recent exposure has documented its presence in many preschools and day-care centers. (*p. 875*)

100–105: Casper has otitis media and needs to been seen. So 100 is **(c)**. The fever theoretically could be a reaction to measles vaccine, but that wouldn't explain his other symptoms. (as an aside, there must be a measles epidemic in your community, since the routine use of vaccine is at 15 months of age.) In 101, if you (incorrectly) chose an antibiotic in 100 or 103, all *except* (b) would be adequate to cover streptococcal, pneumococcal, and *H. influenzae* infection, assuming good physical examination and follow-up. At the ER (103) (a) is the only correct answer. The answer to 104 is (d), based on the URI, sudden fever, and refusal to nurse on the right breast (which you hypothesize increases the pressure on the left tympanic membrane), plus the fact that we made such a big deal about curetting the cerumen. 105 is (b); 2 weeks for the otitis follow-up and 6 months to repeat the measles vaccine.

106. (c); 107. (b) Casper now a has classic case of acute viral laryngotracheitis; the restlessness probably indicates hypoxia. Once the decision is made to intubate, oxygenation is important to provide a margin of safety in case there is difficulty with the procedure. The case is unlikely to be *Hemophilus influenzae* infection because of the proceeding URI for 2 days, similar illness in other family members, and lack of drooling. Allergic croup is generally afebrile, as is a foreign body, and we already told you (in 100), that Casper is immunized, so diphtheria is unlikely.

108. (f) The titer is falling, which in a 4-month-old is consistent with passively acquired maternal antibody (half-life 25 to 28 days). (*p. 795*)

109. (b) The fourfold rise from undetectable levels to presence of antibody indicates infection. The adolescent and adult populations in the United States are the most susceptible age groups. (*p. 792*)

110. (e) The presence of antibody in the acute specimen with a fourfold or greater rise indicates reinfection. There is no viremia and no placental infection. No action is needed. In fact, once an individual is known to be immune, no further titers should be drawn. (*p. 795*)

111. (c) Adenovirus 12 causes a pertussis-like syndrome infrequently. If such a clinical picture accompanied these serologic findings, it would be sufficient evidence. (*p. 816*)

112. (d) Anti-EBNA is antibody to EB virus nucleic acid, and its presence is documentary of past infection. (*pp. 806–807*)

113. (f) The rise in antibody is not significant. The FDA standard rubella antibody serum has varied from 1:256 to 1:2048, depending on the antigen, cells, technician, etc. To document infection, you must be sure both sera are tested together.

114. (c); 115. (g); 116. (e); 117. (a); 118. (b); 119. (d); 120. (f) If you answered all these correctly, you could participate in a trivia contest.

13
The Digestive System

1. **(e)** Both fluoride and tetracycline can lead to brown discoloration. Hyperbilirubinemia will lead to blue-black color. (*p. 924*)

2. **(b); 3. (d)** Caries is most prevalent in children 4 to 8 and 12 to 18 years old. Although fluoridation is considered a Communist plot by some, it is one of the most effective public health measures we have. (*pp. 925–929*)

4. **(d),** which is associated with vitamin deficiency. Surgical "clipping" of the frenum should be done rarely and not until 8 to 10 months of age. (*p. 934*)

5. **(e)** Polyhydramnios would be expected. (*pp. 941–942*)

6. **(d)** Surgery should be attempted only if medical management fails after a 6-week trial or sooner if aspiration pneumonia occurs. The lack of relaxation described in (b) is achalasia and iron deficiency only occurs if there is severe esophagitis. (*pp. 943–945*)

7. **(a)** This problem cannot be treated well. Prevention through childproof caps and parental safety precautions is the best hope. Diptheria is preventible, but not common; peptic esophagitis is common, but not preventable. (*p. 945*)

8. **(c)** If the coin were in the trachea it would be seen on edge in the AP projection. (*p. 946*)

9. **(b) or (d)** The decision as to which procedure to use depends on the experience and availability of the person doing it. (*p. 946*)

10. **(c); 11. (b)** Since the obstruction is proximal to the ampulla of Vater, the vomitus cannot be bile stained, and since most of the vomitus has stomach acid (HCl), one is left with a hypochloremic alkalosis. (*pp. 948–950*)

12. **(e)** There is no such thing as mild atresia (*p. 951*)

13. **(c)** Congenital aganglionic megacolon accounts for 33% of all neonatal obstructions and is the most common colonic obstruction. (*p. 954*)

14. **(c)** Both have lots of stool palpable. (*p. 955, Table 13–3*)

15. **(b)** The usual presentation is painless rectal bleeding. (*p. 956*)

16. **(b)** Some duplications are tubular. (*p. 957*)

17. **(b)** Intussusception does not generally cause an ileus. (*p. 958*)

18. **(a)** If you suggest (b), (c), or (d), the mother will either go elsewhere or call you back in an hour to say things are worse and now he has bloody "jelly-like" stools. (e) is a little hasty and is neither the appropriate time for referral nor the appropriate person to refer the child to.

19. **(d)** The history is classic for intussusception.

20. **(e)** usually works. If it fails, if the symptoms have been present for 48 hours, or if there are signs of obstruction present, then it is time for surgery. (*p. 959*)

21. **(b)** Generally, low lesions have an external fistula. (*pp. 961–962*)

22. **(a)** Cell-mediated immunity is normal, although immunoglobulin levels are low. B_{12} malabsorption is common, and oral fluids may not be tolerated for weeks. (*p. 977*)

23. **(b)** Males are affected more than females after age 6. (*p. 964*)

24. **(c)** Acid secretion has not been shown to be consistently different from controls, gastric ulcers are on the lesser curvature, and the best antacids for children are liquid, not tablets. (*pp. 964–966*)

25. **(e)** Most infections are viral and self-limited. (*pp. 830–832*)

26. **(d)** Greasy stools are found in sprue. (*p. 982*)

27. **(c)** This is a review question from the earlier chapter on neonatal disease, since NEC affects neonates. Bloody stools are found in 25% of cases, medical management fails in 50% of cases when pneumatosis is present,

and breast milk has not been shown to be protective. (*p. 476*)

28. **(c)** Vitamin C is water soluble and is not an indicator of fat malabsorption. (*p. 974*)

29. **(b)** It is D-xylose that is used. (*p. 974*)

30. **(c)** Sucrose is not a reducing sugar. It must be hydrolyzed to be found in a Clinitest exam. (*p. 983*)

31. **(b); 32. (a); 33. (b); 34. (c); 35. (d)** One should not need to call a nutritionist to answer these. (*pp. 983–985*)

36. **(b)** Juvenile pernicious anemia is caused by a lack of intrinsic factor. (*p. 113*)

37. **(a)** Everything can get confused, but Crohn disease is most tricky. Mesenteric adenitis is rare. (*pp. 987–989*)

38. **(d)** Arthritis is found in 10% of patients. Anal fissures are more common in Crohn disease. (*pp. 966–968*)

39. **(b)** Dietary restrictions are unnecessary. (*pp. 967–968*)

40. **(a)** Usually caused by constipation. (*p. 990*)

41. **(c)** Girls have hernias also. (*p. 994*)

42. **(d)** Crigler-Najjar syndrome is a cause of unconjugated hyperbilirubinemia. (*pp. 1013–1015*)

43. **(b)** But to be effective, the Kasai procedure should be performed prior to 2 months of age. (*pp. 1011–1012*)

44. **(d)** This is the more serious form of chronic hepatitis. (*p. 1022*)

45. **(e)** GSD causes massive hepatomegaly but not cirrhosis. (*p. 1029*)

46. **(e)** The liver is shrunken in cirrhosis. (*p. 1029*)

47–50: A classic case of pyloric stenosis is described. The fact that the parents are encountering marital problems needs to be discussed and evaluated, but this is not a cause of failure to thrive nor a cause of rare neurologic disease. Chalasia is unlikely here because of the dropping off of the weight curve and the x-ray findings. Rehydration and correction of alkalosis prior to surgery are important and lead to a better outcome.

47. All except **(e)** are pertinent.

48. **(c)** The ultrasound or upper GI series will be the most productive.

49. **(b)**

50. **(a), (c),** and **(e)**—in that order.

51. **(d)** Urolithiasis pain *is* back pain and is referred to the groin.

52. **(c); 53. (c); 54. (f); 55. (e); 56. (b); 57. (g); 58. (e); 59. (c); 60. (h).**

14

The Respiratory System

1. **(b)** The second period is *pseudo*glandular. (*p. 1035*)

2. **(c)** Surfactant is a mixture of phospholipids and proteins. It appears in the amniotic fluid 6 weeks after synthesis. Although both glucocorticoids and thyroid hormone *increase* synthesis, only glucocorticoids are therapeutic. (*p. 1036*)

3. **(b)** P_{CO_2} is inversely proportional to alveolar ventilation; the V-P ratio varies throughout the lungs; the diffusion conductance for carbon dioxide is higher for CO_2 and O_2 and disease increases the alveolar-arterial P_{O_2} difference. (*p. 1037*)

4. **(c)** The central controller is a brain stem function. The carotid bodies are part of the afferent process. (*pp. 1041–1043*)

5. **(d)**; 6. **(c)**; 7. **(f)**; 8. **(e)**; 9. **(b)**; 10. **(a)** Knowing the indications for these procedures is important. Tuberculosis is best diagnosed by gastric aspirates, or sputum cultures in older children. (*pp. 1046–1049*)

11. **(d)** Postural drainage is of no proven value in asthma, even though it is done at great expense in time and dollars (*pp. 592, 1112*)

12. **(a)** A Pa_{CO_2} of 45 is always worrisome, but in chronic obstruction such as cystic fibrosis, mild hypercapnia may be tolerated for long periods of time. (*pp. 1050, 1114*)

13. **(d)** The most common form of trauma is probably nose-picking, although admissions are hard to come by. (*p. 1054*)

14. **(a)** The frontal sinuses are not present at age 4. (*pp. 1059–1060*)

15. **(b)** Polyps which are easily distinguished from turbinates cause mucopurulent rhinorrhea, not epistaxis; steroids and decongestants are of little value. (*p. 1060*)

16. **(c)**, **(d)** Tonsillectomy is also indicated for carcinoma of the tonsil. Adenoidectomy may be useful for (e). (*pp. 1060–1061*)

17. **(d)** Acute nasopharyngitis is more severe in children; rhinoviruses are responsible for a third of infections (although strep is the most common bacterial infection). Most children have 5 to 8 infections a year in the first 2 years of life (more if they are in day care) and antibiotics are not useful in reducing incidence of complications. (*p. 1055*)

18. **(e)** Rhinovirus is a cause of acute, not chronic, rhinitis. (*p. 1058*)

19. **(b)** Laryngomalacia will be of great concern to parents who are light sleepers. (b) in the dedication of this book suffered this syndrome. (*pp. 1062–1063*)

20. **(c)** *H. influenzae*, type B causes epiglottitis; type C is not associated with croup. (*pp. 1065–1066*)

21. **(e)** Steroids are of no proven value in croup, although they also do no harm. (*pp. 1067–1068*)

22. **(b)**; 23. **(b)**; 24. **(b)**; 25. **(c)** With a toxic child, admission is reasonable, and blood culture offers the best chance of diagnosis. Ampicillin (or cefuroxime; if resistance is a problem) is a resonable drug of choice, since *Haemophilus influenzae* is a not uncommon etiology for pneumonia in 2-year-olds. The recurrence, however, is the tip-off that there is something else going on, and in this age group a foreign body is common—thus the need for an inspiratory-expiratory film study. (*pp. 1069–1071*)

26. **(a)** RSV is the etiologic agent for bronchiolitis; influenza virus causes croup. (*p. 1075*)

27. **(b)** Bacterial infection occurs rarely as pneumonia, occasionally as acute bronchitis. The pneumococcus is the usual etiologic agent. 3 to 5% mortality occurred before the advent of antibiotics. (*pp. 1077–1080*)

28. **(c)** Infants are most susceptible to staph pneumonia. (*pp. 1079–1081*)

29. **(e)** Hamman-Rich syndrome causes alveolar-capillary block and fibrosis, not atelectasis. (*pp. 1092–1094*)

30. **(a)** Left ventricular failure—not right—would cause pulmonary edema. (*p. 1097*)

31. **(a)** The aspirated material generally lodges in the dependent portions of the lung. Anaerobic streptococci and *Fusobacterium* are common pathogens. (*p. 1100*)

32. **(b)** Malignancy is the second leading cause. Tuberculosis is less prevalent, but still causes effusions when it is present. (*p. 1116*)

33. **(c)** **(a)** and **(b)** are not sudden in onset, and **(d)**, staphylococcal pneumonia, is not likely in a healthy adolescent. Aspiration **(e)** is possible but less likely in this age group and even less likely in the left bronchus. (*p. 1118*)

34. **(c)** Pectus looks worse than it is. It rarely needs treatment and rarely causes anything more than cosmetic problems. (*pp. 1120–1121*)

35. **(e)**; 36. **(b)** and **(c)**; 37. **(d)** This case sounds like allergic reactive airway disease, perhaps even a first attack of asthma. The family history, lack of evidence for chronic disease, nocturnal symptoms, and wheezes, all point to that diagnosis. (*pp. 1102–1104*)

38. **(a)**; 39. **(c)**; 40. **(a)** The type of cough is often helpful in diagnosis, but does not substitute for x-ray and/or laboratory confirmation. (*p. 1103—Table 14–4*)

15

The Cardiovascular System

1. **(b)** is correct. An apical heave occurs with left ventricular hypertrophy. (*p. 1131*)

2. **(c)** (b) would be a venous hum and (d) an innocent pulmonic murmur. A Still murmur is most common between 3 and 7 years of age, so (e) is incorrect, and it is innocent, so (a) is also wrong. This edition of the textbook describes the murmur, but does not name it. (*p. 1132*)

3. **(e)** The ECG looks different in a premature infant but is not useful in diagnosis. (*pp. 1133–1135*)

4. **(c); 5. (a); 6. (a); 7. (b); 8. (a); 9. (c); 10. (b)** Tall P waves are associated with right atrial hypertrophy and flattened waves with left atrial enlargement. (*p. 1135*)

11. **(a)** Figure 15–32 on page 1145 depicts this clearly.

12. **(c)** m mode is for morphology; Doeppler for flow. In some cases (e.g., PDA) no cath is required prior to surgery. Transesophageal echo is excellent for atrial lesions. (*pp. 1137–1138*)

13. **(a)** Children born in 1965 in the United States were the last large risk group following the epidemic of 1964. This is now a problem for internists to deal with. (*pp. 1173, 1177*)

14. **(b)** VSDs are most common in infants and children. In older children and adults, ASD, PDA, tetralogy, and pulmonary stenosis are as common as VSD. (*p. 1147, Table 15–6*)

15. **(c)** The four components of the tetralogy are pulmonary stenosis, ventricular septal defect, dextroposition of the aorta, and right ventricular hypertrophy. (*p. 1149*)

16. **(e)** More males than females are affected. (*pp. 1156–1157*)

17. **(a)** Echocardiography has improved diagnosis but not treatment. The surgical procedures (c) and (d) are for treatment of tetralogy. Home oxygen availability is palliative only. (*p. 1157*)

18. **(d)** The second sound is single. (*p. 1154*)

19. **(c)** 30–50% of small VSDs close spontaneously. (*pp. 1167–1168*)

20. **(c)** The flow through an atrial septal defect is not under sufficient pressure to create a murmur. The second sound is fixed in its split, not variable; the defect is either ostium primum or ostium secundum, not a patent foramen ovale; and heart failure is rare. (*pp. 1169–1172*)

21. **(c)** Children with ostium primum are often asymptomatic; ostium secundum is well tolerated in childhood. When the A-V canal and cushion defect are present, trouble begins early. (*p. 1171*)

22. **(a)** As the pulmonary pressure increases and approaches the systemic pressure, backflow is decreased and the diastolic murmur disappears. (*p. 1173*)

23. **(d)** 98% are just below the left subclavian. (*p. 1177*)

24. **(c)** The notching is caused by increased collateral arteries trying to supply the lower trunk and extremities. (*p. 1178*)

25. **(b)** The left superior vena cava is the site of 40% of cases. The next most common sites are coronary sinus (20%), right atrium (20%), and right superior vena cava (10%). (*p. 1159—Table 15–8*)

26. **(a)** Of all the aortic stenosis syndromes, supravalvular type is rare but is the only type associated with the features mentioned. (*pp. 1180–1181*)

27. **(e)** is correct and shows supraventricular tachycardia. (a) is sinus arrhythmia with junctional escape beats (2 and 9); (b) is atrial fibrillation; (c) shows premature atrial contractions; and (d) shows premature ventricular contractions. None of these would give the stated symptom. (*pp. 1193–1195*)

28. **(a)** In infants (b) would be used because of a high rate of recurrence. (*p. 1195*)

29. **(a)** Rheumatic heart disease used to be the most common underlying factor, but congenital heart disease is now the prime etiol-

ogy. Dental surgery is a secondary factor. (*p. 1200*)

30. **(d)** The critical laboratory test is the blood culture. All others are secondary. (*p. 1201*)

31. **(a)** occurs first. (b) or (d) may follow after a number of years. (c) and (e) are less common. (*p. 1204*)

32. **(c)** The P-R interval is increased, not decreased, with digitalization. (*p. 1214*)

33. **(a)** Paradoxical pulse is also seen in the blood culture. All others are secondary. (*p. 1218*)

34. **(c)** This is rare, but the absence of a cardiac murmur and the presence of the cranial bruit imply high output failure. (*p. 1220*)

35. **(c)** is incurable, although transplantation may be available. (*pp. 1223–1224, 1346*)

36–37. These problems concern the diagnosis and management of hypertension. In 36 all of the responses are needed (plus others, no doubt) *except* (b), which is not particularly pertinent. Even though the oral contraceptives may be causing this patient's mild hypertension, confirmation of the elevation is necessary before any work-up, making **(a)** the answer to 37. If the 140/100 level is confirmed, then (d) would be appropriate (after counseling as to other birth control measures). If this failed to reduce the blood pressure over the next year, then a work-up would be in order. (e) is just not warranted at this blood pressure level. (*pp. 1225–1227*)

38. **(b)** Most newborns with hypertension usually have an umbilical arterial catheter in place, or a renal problem. (*p. 1223*)

39. **(e)** Along with rhabdomyomas and fibromas, myxomas are the most common of otherwise rare events. A rhabdomyosarcoma (or any malignant tumor is rarer still, generally appearing every 4 to 5 years in CPCs. (*p. 1221*)

40. **(e)**; 41. **(c)**; 42. **(a)**; 43. **(b)**; 44. **(d)**; 45. **(a)** All these are antihypertensives with differing dosage forms, routes of administration, and side effects. If you have them memorized, that's fine, but before administering or ordering them, it's wise to read the package insert of Physicians Desk Reference (PDR). (*p. 1226—Table 15–25*)

16

Diseases of the Blood

1. **(c)** Hb F constitutes 70% of total hemoglobin at birth. (*p. 1230*)

2. **(d)** Heme iron needs to be in the ferrous form. (*p. 1231*)

3. **(d)** "Physiologic" anemia occurs at 3 months. (*p. 1232—Table 16–2*)

4. **(b)** Erythropoietin activity is low although levels are high. (*pp. 1232–1233*)

5. **(a)** Goat's milk is deficient in folic acid. (*pp. 1236–1239*)

6. **(b)** Chronic blood loss would lead to iron deficiency and microcytosis. (a) leads to malabsorption of folic acid, (c) causes a 25% increase in the need for folic acid, (d) is a B_{12} deficiency, and (e) is a primary blocker of folate activity. (*p. 1237, Fig. 16–3*)

7. **(c)** This mechanism is related to neither lactase deficiency nor milk "allergy." Substitution of heated or evaporated cow's milk or reduction of intake to less than 1 pint/day will prevent the problem. (*p. 1239*)

8. **(a), (b), and (c)** Sickle cell anemia is a hemoglobinopathy. (*pp. 1245–1247*)

9. **(a) and (c)** The inheritance pattern is X-linked, and the diagnostic level of activity is 10% or less of normal. (*pp. 1245–1246*)

10. **(a) and (c)** Sequestration occurs only in children; the slide test is rapid but not precise. Hemoglobin electrophoresis is needed for conclusive diagnosis. (*pp. 1247–1250*)

11. **(d)** Sickle trait, thalassemia minor, and hemoglobin-C thalassemia are mild. Sickle cell disease does not cause the symptoms described. (*pp. 1250–1254*)

12. **(c)** Dehydration causes hemoconcentration but not polycythemia. (*p. 1257*)

13. **(a)** Bone marrow transplantation can also be tried in histocompatible donors. (*p. 1258*)

14. **(T)** Obvious. (*p. 1260*)

15. **(F)** Not unless there are symptoms of clinical distress. (*p. 1260*)

16. **(F)** There are few problems from incompatible platelets, but some RBCs travel with them, so compatibility (esp. Rh) is desirable. (*p. 1260*)

17. **(F)** Testing is not possible for other viral forms of hepatitis. (*p. 1261*)

18. **(T)** The urticaria is easily treated. Transfusion can continue. (*p. 1262*)

19. **(T)** The patient with chronic anemia is usually well compensated. (*p. 1260*)

20. **(F)** There is too low a concentration of WBCs, and they die quickly. (*p. 1260*)

21. **(b)** Not to be confused with the white cell count, which includes lymphocytes, eosinophils, etc. (*p. 1264*)

22. **(a)** Stress causes a mobilization of white cells into the blood stream and in an increased white cell count. (*p. 1265*)

23. **(c)** The number of neutrophils and their ability to increase in numbers are normal. The WBCs cannot reduce NBT. (*pp. 1269–1270*)

24. **(a)** Factor VII is part of the extrinsic system. (*p. 1273*)

25. **(d)** Fresh frozen plasma or cryoprecipitate (concentrate of factor VIII) is therapeutic. (*pp. 1275–1276*)

26. **(b)** The prothrombin time measures factors II, V, VII, and X. (*p. 1274*)

27. **(b); 28. (c); 29. (d); 30. (e)** Hemophilia A is "classic," B is Christmas disease, C is plasma thromboplastin antecedent deficiency, and the Hageman factor has no other name. (*pp. 1275–1277*)

31. **(b)** Breast milk is deficient in vitamin K, and if a broad-spectrum antibiotic is given to the infant, the bowel flora may not synthesize the vitamin, leading to disaster. (*pp. 486–487*)

32. **(a)** This is a classic case of iron-deficiency anemia, undoubtedly nutritional in origin. Pica is a common symptom and makes lead

poisoning possible but not the most likely diagnosis. (*p. 1239*)

33. **(b)** Reticulocytosis peaks at 5 to 7 days. (*p. 1240*)

34. **(c)** Stores of iron need to be repleted, and 4 to 8 weeks does it. (*p. 1240*)

35. **(a), (b),** and **(e)** Sickle cell anemia is not seen in Caucasians, and UTI is highly unlikely in an otherwise healthy boy. (*p. 1239*)

36. **(d)** Ivemark syndrome includes dextrocardia. (*p. 1288*)

37. **(c)** and **(d)** Pneumococci are the leading cause of sepsis, and infants rather than older children are at greater risk. Those with spherocytosis are at lower risk than those with thalassemia, lipidosis, or immune-deficiency diseases. (*p. 1288*)

38–45. (*pp. 1280–1283*)

38. **(b)** A purpura, but with normal counts.

39. **(b)** Adhesiveness is impaired.

40. **(a)** Idiopathic thrombocytopenic purpura, obviously.

41. **(a)** Also eczema and immune deficiency.

42. **(c)** Thrombocytosis is common.

43. **(a)** Platelets are consumed along with the factors.

44. **(a)** The name gives the answer again.

45. **(a)** On the basis of trapping of the platelets in the cavernous hemangioma.

46. **(e); 47. (b); 48. (c); 49. (d); 50. (a)** See Table 16–13 and pp. 1277–1279 for all these answers. Most of the time, a hematologist will be available to do and sort out these tests.

17

Neoplasms and Neoplasm-Like Lesions

1. **(c)** Cancer causes more deaths than any other disease, but unintentional injury is the leading cause of death in children. (*p. 1291*)

2. **(d); 3. (c); 4. (c); 5. (b); 6. (e); 7. (f); 8. (a); 9. (d); 10. (c)** These are relatively rare conditions, but their genetic link sets them apart. (*pp. 1292–1293. See also Table 7–8, pp. 288–289*)

11. **(d); 12. (c); 13. (a); 14. (c); 15. (b); 16. (f); 17. (c); 18. (d); 19. (a); 20. (b)** The mechanisms of action and toxicities of the various chemotherapeutic agents are listed in Table 17–2. (*p. 1295*)

21. **(d)** If you answered this correctly you either guessed, have had good electives in hematology, or are a hematologist.

22. **(b)** This figure depicts rosette formation with sheep erythrocytes. It is diagnostic of T-cell ALL. (Rosette formation is also seen in neuroblastoma but sheep cells are not necessary to see this formation.)

23. **(d)** The B-cell form has the worst prognosis of the first three choices followed by the T-cell form. The best prognosis is null cell. (e) is now false. (*p. 1299*)

24. **(e)** There is also an increased frequency of Hodgkin disease in the 50+ age group. (*p. 1301*)

25. **(c)** The cell is a Reed-Sternberg cell, which is diagnostic of Hodgkin disease. (*p. 1301*)

26. **(d)** The younger the infant, the better the prognosis. (*p. 1304–1307*)

27. **(a)** So are hemihypertrophy and sporadic aniridia. (*p. 1307*)

28. **(c)** Rhabdomyosarcoma accounts for more than half the soft tissue sarcomas. (*p. 1309*)

29. **(d)** Amputation is not the treatment of choice for Ewing sarcoma. (*pp. 1311–1314, Table 17–12*)

30. **(d)** Also known as lymphoepithelioma. (*p. 1316*)

31. **(c)** If stress fractures occur, curettage may be necessary, but is not usual. (*pp. 1319–1320*)

32. **(b)** Leukokoria is also seen in retinal detachment, persistent hyperplastic primary vitreous, visceral larva migrans, bacterial panendophthalmitis, cataract, coloboma of the choroid, and retinopathy of prematurity. (*p. 1314*)

33. **(c)** Teratomas or teratocarcinomas fit the description best. (*pp. 1317–1318*)

34. **(C)** Both are benign. (*p. 1320*)

35. **(A)** Hemangiomas may cause high output failure. (*p. 1320*)

36. **(B)** Surgery, not steroids, is indicated in lymphangioma. (*p. 1320*)

37. **(A)** Steroids, not surgery, are indicated in hemangioma. (*p. 1320*)

38. **(B)** The skin is the more common site for hemangioma. (*p. 1320*)

39. **(C)** Since both may occur in the head and neck, obstruction can occur. (*p. 1320*)

40. **(D)** Both tumors affect infants most commonly. (*p. 1320*)

18

The Urinary System and Pediatric Gynecology

1. **(b)** The juxtaglomerular apparatus is part of the blood supply to nephrons. (*pp. 1323–1324*)

2. **(a)** UV/P also measures GFR is solute is freely filtered through the glomerulus. (*p. 1325*)

3. **(c)** Homogentisic acid colors the urine black. (*p. 1326*)

4. **(d)** Hypercalciuria causes hematuria, but not from glomerular damage. (*pp. 1326—Table 18–2*)

5. **(b)** Immunologic injury is the most common cause for glomerulonephritis (*p. 1326*)

6. **(a)** IgA is predominant. (*p. 1328*)

7. **(d)** Pharyngitis-associated AGN is a winter illness, is more common in boys, and follows strep 10 to 15% of the time. Second attacks are rare. (*pp. 1329–1331*)

8. **(b)** Hyponatremia, as a result of volume overload, is more common. (*p. 1331*)

9. **(e)** The serum C3 level is normal in anaphylactoid purpura. (*pp. 1331–1335*)

10. **(c)** The name gives the answer away. (*p. 1335*)

11. **(a), (b), (c)** Plasma lipoproteins are increased. (*pp. 1340–1343*)

12. **(b), (d)** Complement levels and blood pressure are usually normal. (*p. 1341*)

13. **(c), (d), (e)** Fever and exercise are non-pathologic causes of hematuria (*pp. 1338–1340, Table 18–4*)

14. **(a)** Prednisone at 60 mg/m²/24 hrs. is safe, effective, and relatively inexpensive. The others should be used if steroids fail. (*p. 1342*)

15. **(c)** Type 12 with pharyngitis; type 49 with pyoderma. This piece of trivia was deleted from this edition of the Textbook.

16. **(B)**; 17. **(M)**; 18. **(D)**; 19. **(P)**; 20. **(D)**; 21. **(P)**; 22. **(D)**; 23. **(P)**; 24. **(P)** I am not sure these distinctions need to be memorized as long as the possibility is kept in mind that they do occur. (*p. 1346—Table 18–5*)

25. **(a), (c), (e)** Vasopressin does not increase urine osmolality in nephrogenic DI, and unlimited access to water is most important. (*pp. 1347–1348*)

26. **(a), (c), (d)** In distal RTA polyuria may occur with failure to thrive, but polydipsia is not a cardinal symptom. Renal glycosuria is benign and symptomless.

27. **(a), (b), (e)** Prognosis is uncertain. Many patients do well. Infants present with growth failure, older children with muscle weakness or carpel-pedal spasm. (*p. 1348*)

28. **(d)** The other choices do not have significant hepatic disease. (*p. 1337*)

29. **(d)** Congenital renal obstruction generally causes renal failure in the newborn period and is postrenal. The others are renal causes. (*p. 1352—Table 18–9*)

30. **(b), (c), (e)** Serum potassium and phosphorus are elevated in acute renal failure. (*p. 1353*)

31. **(e)** Methanol intoxication must be treated with hemodialysis. (*pp. 1358, 1776*)

32. **(a), (b), (d)** Infants with CRF usually have congenital abnormalities, which are three times more common in males than in females. (*pp. 1355–1356*)

33. **(b), (c), (d), (e)** Hyperglycemia follows an oral glucose load in CRF. (*p. 1356, Table 18–10*)

34. **(a), (b), (c), (d), (e)** All drugs listed must be given in reduced dosage in children with renal failure. It is wise to read package inserts on all drugs before giving them. (*p. 1358*)

35. **(b)**, **(d)**, **(e)** Frequency, urgency, and dysuria may indicate cystitis or urethritis without renal involvement. Red cell casts are not present. (*pp. 1360–1363*)

36. **(a)**, **(b)**, **(e)** Gonadotropins are normal, and associated urinary anomalies are uncommon. (*pp. 1378–1379*)

37. **(a)**, **(c)**, **(e)**. The most common stone is calcium *oxalate*, not carbonate. Lithotriptors are terrific, and make surgery a thing of the past, but treatment of the underlying disorder is also required. (*pp. 1381–1382*)

38. **(a)**, **(b)**, **(c)**, **(d)** Herpes generally causes ulcerations, not vaginitis. Any of these (except bubble bath) may be acquired as a result of sexual abuse. (*pp. 1384–1386*)

39. **(a)**, **(b)**, **(c)**, **(d)**, **(e)** All of these can cause prepubertal vaginal bleeding, as can sexual abuse. (*pp. 1384–1392*)

40. **(a)**, **(b)**, **(e)** DES, not viruses, is associated with adenocarcinoma of the vagina. Unfortunately, the Pap smear is less reliable in adenocarcinoma of the vagina than in carcinoma of the cervix (but it should still be done). (*pp. 1391–1392*)

41. **(d)** The abdominal mass is likely to be hydronephrosis. (*p. 1368*)

42. **(e)** Torsions and epididymitis are painful. Hydroceles are smooth. (*pp. 1379–1380*)

43. **(b)** Adenocarcinoma is very rare. Thus, mammography is not indicated in adolescents. Fat necrosis is usually secondary to trauma. (*p. 1389*)

44. **(a)** Reassurance is appropriate at age 15. Work-up should be begun after 16 years of age. (*p. 537*)

45–50. This is a case of acute urinary tract infection in a young girl. In 45, **(a)**, **(b)**, **(c)**, and **(e)** are correct. Fever will help determine whether upper or lower tract disease is present. Bubble bath will cause urethritis, as will pinworms. (d) is more likely in glomerulonephritis, which does not present with this history. In the work-up (46), **(b)** and **(c)** are the crucial tests, and in 47 the most likely diagnosis is lower urinary tract infection **(b)**. The presence of white cells and bacteria rules out benign familial hematuria. **(b)** is best in 48, although some would use (d) or oral ampicillin or other drugs (not choices here). The key in 49 is **(a)**, *follow-up*. Some would argue for (b) as well, but good people differ in opinion regarding whether to do radiographs in first or second UTIs in young girls. (c), (d), and (e) are not appropriate. The IVP (50) shows reflux and a diverticulum (d) for which surgery is required.

19

The Endocrine System

1. **(a), (b), (e)** Pituitary hormones act on other cells. TSH is inhibited by thyroxine and triiodothyronine. No hypothalamic inhibitor is known for thyrotropin. (*pp. 1397–1398*)

2. **(a)** The *most* common cause of hypothyroidism is thyroiditis, but of the choices given, craniopharyngioma is first. (*p. 1398*)

3. **(b)** Growth hormone levels increase with sleep and are stimulated by L-dopa and exercise. (*p. 1401*)

4. **(c); 5. (b)** These children have adequate growth potential. If chronologic age and skeletal maturation were similar, genetic short stature would be present. (*p. 1402*)

6. **(d)** Removing the child to a stimulating environment will stimulate growth. (*p. 1402*)

7. **(a), (b)** Also frontal bossing, small triangular facies, sparse subcutaneous tissue, and clinodactyly. (*p. 1402*)

8. **(e)** Amelioration of symptoms often indicates that the tumor has progressed into the anterior pituitary. (*p. 1403*)

9. **(b)** The sodium levels are depressed because water is not excreted. Restricting fluids and capitalizing on the insensible loss is therapeutic. (*p. 1405*)

10. **(a), (b), (d)** Children with precocious puberty are taller as children; the others catch up as adults. Provera has too many adverse effects to be used therapeutically. The treatment of choice is an LH-RH analog. (*pp. 1408–1409*)

11. **(b), (c), (d)** Thyroxine does not cross the placenta. Thyroiditis is the most common etiology of acquired hypothyroidism. (*pp. 1416–1418, 1420*)

12. **(b), (d), (e)** Girls are affected more often than boys, and bone age is retarded at birth. (*pp. 1417–1420*)

13. **(a), (d), (e)** Iodine-deficiency goiter is no longer seen in the United States, and goiter may occur in euthyroid children. (*pp. 1423–1425*)

14. **(b), (c)** A positive titer rules in lymphocytic thyroiditis. TSH levels are normal in simple goiter and are elevated in thyroiditis. (*pp. 1421–1422*)

15. **(d)** The names of these signs are Graefe (upper eyelid lag), Moebius (inability to converge), and Stellwag (retraction of the eyelid). (*p. 1426*)

16. **(b), (c), (d), (e)** Boys are affected as often as girls, since the disease is stimulated by maternal factors. (*p. 1427*)

17. **(c), (d), (e)** A sudden enlargement of a nodule present for years is probably hemorrhage. A "cold" nodule should be watched unless it meets the other listed criteria. (*p. 1428*)

18. **(c)** Calcium may be needed immediately, but vitamin D_2 is maintenance. (*pp. 1433–1434*)

19. **(b)** Parathyroid hormone is elevated. (*p. 1436*)

20. **(e)** Tuberculosis used to be first, but no longer. The others are found in adults. (*p. 1441*)

21. **(a); 22. (a) and (b)** This is a case of Addison disease, and replacement therapy with both DOCA and hydrocortisone is necessary. (*p. 1444*)

23. **(d)** It accounts for 95% of all cases of congenital adrenal hyperplasia. (*pp. 1444–1445*)

24. **(a), (b), (c), (e)** Urinary 17-ketosteroids are usually increased. (*p. 1448*)

25. **(c)** Sipple syndrome includes pheochromocytoma and medullary carcinoma of the thyroid. (*pp. 1452, 1686*)

26. **(b)** Gynecomastia is pathologic in young children and is usually caused by exogenous estrogen. (*p. 1459*)

27. **(d)** Hypertension is not part of the syndrome (*p. 1463*)

28. **(a)** These patients may have mental retardation, but gonadal function is normal (*p. 1462*)

29. **(a)** Swyer syndrome is an example of male pseudohermaphroditism. (*p. 1465*)

30. **(a), (b), (d), (e)** Noonan syndrome can occur in males and females. (*p. 1462*)

20

Neurologic and Muscular Disorders

1. **(b)**, **(c)** Infections are generally etiologic in the first 2 years of life. In the neonatal period, anoxia, congenital anomalies, and hemorrhage are most common. Idiopathic epilepsy leads in midchildhood and adolescence. (*pp. 1491–1499*)

2. **(b)**, **(d)**, **(e)** The occurrence of grand mal seizures in newborns is unusual, and the prognosis is better than one would think. (*pp. 1500–1501*)

3. **(a)**, **(c)** The EEG may remain abnormal for weeks, seizures with *Shigella* rarely recur, and one recurrence is not worrisome. (*pp. 1495–1496*)

4. **(b)** Petit mal seizures start after 3 years of age and may end by puberty. Girls are affected more often than boys. (*p. 1493*)

5. **(a)**, **(b)** The other waves are normal. (*p. 1481*)

6. **(b)**, **(d)** The most common cause is failure to take medication; 1 to 2 mg/kg of phenobarbital is too little; and inhalation anesthesia is a last resort. (*pp. 1501–1503*)

7. **(c)** Some precautions are necessary (e.g., no swimming alone). (*pp. 1496–1499*)

8. **(a)**, **(c)** Sodium valproate causes nausea and alopecia, not sedation, and is not as successful in controlling psychomotor seizures as the other drugs. (*p. 1498*)

9. **(a)**; 10. **(a)**; 11. **(c)**; 12. **(a) and (c)**; 13. **(b)**; 14. **(b)**; 15. **(a) and (b)**; 16. **(d)** These therapeutic agents have their own dosage schedule, toxicity, and indications. New is not always better. (*pp. 1496–1499—Table 20–5*)

17. **All are true.** Most children with epilepsy lead normal useful lives. (*p. 1498*)

18. **(b)**, **(d)** Strength and coordination are decreased. There are no involuntary movements. (*pp. 1477–1478*)

19. **(b)**, **(c)**, **(d)** Basal ganglia lesions cause chorea, cerebellar lesions lead to intention tremors, and fasciculations occur in anterior horn disease. (*pp. 1478–1479*)

20. **(b)** It is usually a craniopharyngioma that presses on the optic chiasm. (*p. 1476*)

21. **(d)**, **(e)** Moro, placing, and stepping reflexes are normally gone by 4 months. (*p. 1479*)

22. **(d)**; 23. **(b)**; 24. **(a)**; 25. **(b)**; 26. **(d)**; 27. **(b)**; 28. **(b)** The differential diagnosis of coma is important clinically. A table represents a nice way of approaching the problem. (*pp. 1518–1520—Table 20–9*)

29. **(b)**, **(c)**, **(d)** The anomaly usually occurs at L5 to S1, and lipomas, not dermoids, are present in 40% of cases (*p. 1483*)

30. **(a)**, **(d)** Communicating hydrocephalus can also follow infection and subarachnoid hemorrhage and accompanies Hurler syndrome, achondroplasia, and vitamin A intoxication. (*p. 1489*)

31. **(c)** Anoxia is the leading cause of CP, and spastic CP is the most common type. (*p. 1515*)

32. **(a)**, **(b)**, **(d)** Laboratory studies are not helpful, and phenobarbital is not useful for long-term therapy. (*pp. 1506–1529*)

33. **(c)** Tuberous sclerosis is autosomal dominant and a major cause of mental retardation. (*p. 1510*)

34. **(a)**, **(e)** The other three are diseases of the white matter. (*pp. 1524–1529*)

35. **(d)** MS is rare in children (less than 1% of cases appear before 15 years of age) but with pediatrics caring for older and older children, this is worth knowing. (*p. 1528*)

36. **(b)** There is a decrease or absence of IgA and IgE and delayed hypersensitivity. (*pp. 1512–1513*)

37. (a); 38 (a) This does sound like the presentation of a tumor. The hypotonia of the arm and leg (a focal sign) makes the other choices unlikely. An astrocytoma is the most common finding at this age given the choices (medulloblastoma is the other). (*p. 1532*)

39. (a), (b), (c), (e) The incidence of Reye syndrome has dropped markedly since the recognition of the link to asperin; phenothiazines are never indicated. (*pp. 1020–1021*)

40. (b), (d), (e) The chapter avoids telling you that the *most* common cause of acute and chronic subdural hematomas is child abuse. You should not forget that, nor should you avoid the issue. (Also, the references are dated and misleading.) (*pp. 1521–1523*)

41. (c), (d) Urinary VMA is low, HVA is high, and the pressor response is exaggerated. (*pp. 1557–1558*)

42. (a), (b) Guillain-Barré syndrome affects peripheral nerves and nerve roots, Riley-Day autonomic nerves, and atonic diplegia is cortical. (*pp. 1555–1556*)

43. (c) Poliomyelitis is asymmetric. Coxsackievirus infection may precede Guillain-Barré syndrome, but it is usually over by the time paralysis begins. (*p. 1558*)

44. (b) In this case secondary to herpes zoster. (*p. 1559*)

45. (e) She has myasthenia gravis. (*p. 1554*)

46. (a), (c), (e) This is congenital torticollis. It is caused by hemorrhage into the sternocleidomastoid muscle, not by a tumor or myositis, so (b) and (d) are incorrect. (*p. 1544*)

47. (c) Duchenne muscular dystrophy is also called pseudohypertrophic muscular dystrophy. (*pp. 1544–1545*)

48–50: (c), (a), (b) Most of the other disorders in this chapter are beyond help. The treatment of these disorders is discussed in the last edition of the Textbook. (*pp. 1548–1550*)

21

Disorders of the Eye and Ear

1. (c), (d) The blue color is normal in newborns. The lens is more spherical, and, even though acuity is about 20/400, newborns can fixate on their parents' eyes at birth. (*p. 1561*)

2. (a) Most newborns are hyperopic, but this will vary according to the size of the eye, the state of the lens, and the curvature of the cornea. (*p. 1561*)

3. (c), (d), (e) The image falls anterior to the retina, and the far point of clear vision varies inversely with the degree of myopia. (*p. 1564*)

4. (a), (b), (c) Amblyopia occurs when there is a problem with one eye. (*p. 1565*)

5. (c), (d) Nyctalopia (night blindness), amaurosis (blindness) since birth, and dyslexia are not emergencies. The sudden onset of diplopia or amaurosis implies tumor and must be promptly evaluated. (*pp. 1565–1566*)

6. (b) Diplopia is probable, and the answer to Question 5 applies. (*p. 1566*)

7. (a), (c) The Hirschberg test is negative in pseudostrabismus owing to epicanthal folds. The deviating eye moves out when the fixating eye is covered. (*p. 1570*)

8. (a), (c) Both congenital ptosis and entropion (inversion of the lid margin) are amenable to surgical treatment. (*pp. 1573–1574*)

9. (b) Dacryocystitis neonatorum is quite common. Dacryoadenitis is not. (*p. 1575*)

10. (b) The *most* common cause is silver nitrate, but that was not a choice here. Of the organisms listed, *Chlamydia* is more common, though less serious than *Neisseria gonorrhoeae*. (*pp. 1575–1576*)

11. (b) The fundus depicts chorioretinitis. (*p. 1587*)

12. (a) The problem is immaturity and hyperoxia. (*pp. 1587–1589*)

13. (c), (d) This is a retinoblastoma, which occurs in infants, is usually unilateral, and is not associated with CMV. (*p. 1589*)

14. (d) The fundus depicts hypertensive retinopathy. If present, we should look for a renal disease, pheochromocytoma, coarctation of the aorta, or collagen-vascular disease. (*p. 1592*)

15. (a), (c), (e) The etiology may also be by direct extension of bacteremia. The organisms are generally *Staphylococcus*, *Streptococcus* (β group A and pneumonia), and *Haemophilus*. Treat accordingly and systemically, not topically. (*p. 1597*)

16. (c) These are retinal hemorrhages, which are pathognomonic of child abuse in this age group. (*p. 1599*)

17. (a) Hydrocortisone will make things worse.

18. (b); 19. (d); 20. (e); 21. (f); 22. (a); 23. (d); 24. (c); 25. (a) There are relatively few disorders that cannot be discovered with the ophthalmoscope. (*pp. 1580–1586—Table 22–1*)

26. (c) Hearing loss affects 2/1000 children by age 6, not 2%; it is both peripheral and central in origin; most familial sensorineural hearing loss is autosomal recessive (70 to 80%); and only 6% of hearing impaired children are profoundly so. (*pp. 1602–1603*)

27. (d) Neonatal otitis is an acute infection. While screening is useful in recurrent or chronic otitis, it is not automatically a criterion for neonatal screening. In addition to those listed in (a), (b), (c), and (e), birth weight < 1.5 kg, a positive family history of hearing loss, and craniofacial defects (e.g., submucous cleft palate) should trigger a request for hearing screening. (*p. 1603—Table 22–2*)

28. (B); 29. (C); 30. (A) These are tympanograms. (a) is normal; (b) is from a child with serous otitis media. Sensorineural hearing loss should not affect the tympanogram. (*pp. 1606–1607*)

31. (b) ABR is unaffected by general anesthesia. (*p. 1607*)

32. (a) An interesting fact! The middle and external ears arise from the 1-2 branchial arch; anotia is rare (it is the absence of a pinna; pit depressions only need surgery if they get infected, and inner ear malformations are rare. (*p. 1608*)

33. (d) Pseudomonas is most common. (*p. 1608*)

34. (b); 35. (d); 36. (a); 37. (f); 38. (c); 39. (c) If hemophilis influenza had been listed, it too could have been the correct answer to questions 38 and 39, since Bullous myringitis is not known to be different from acute otitis in etiologic agents. There was a time when we thought mycoplasma were responsible for Bullous otitis media. Note: (b) would be acceptable for 36 also. (*p. 1608–1611*)

40. (b) Traumatic perforations are generally found in the anterior portion of the pars tensa when caused by compression and generally heal spontaneously without the need for tympanoplasty or antibiotics, topical or systemic. (*p. 1618*)

22

Bones, Joints, and Skin

1. **(b)** Metatarsus varus is, with tibal torsion, very common as an etiology for in-toeing. (*p. 1695*)

2. **(b)** Of the choices given, stretching is the best choice, both therapeutically and economically, but if the condition persists, casting may be required. (*p. 1695*)

3. **(a), (b)** The third component is metatarsus varus. (*pp. 1694–1695*)

4. **(d)** If this fails, then surgery is required. (*p. 1694*)

5. **(a)** The vertical talus is the most severe and serious form of flat foot. (*p. 1693*)

6. **(a)** Surgery is only rarely needed, casting is not indicated, and "Thomas heels" do little. (*p. 1693*)

7. **(b), (c), (d)** Calcaneovalgus is a form of club-fllot; lateral femoral anteversion leads to "out-toeing." (*pp. 1697–1698*)

8. **(e)** In-toeing resolves spontaneously. Exercises are a waste of time, orthopedic shoes are a waste of money, and going to the orthopedic surgeon for this problem is both. (*p. 1698*)

9. **(d)** The purpose of shoes is to protect the feet from sharp objects and cold tempertures. Sneakers are fine any time, and high-top and orthopedic shoes are unnecessary and expensive. (*p. 1696*)

10. **(d)** Traction is crucial to stretch the muscles before operation. (*pp. 1707–1708*)

11. **(b)** Infection is first in both age groups. Transient synovitis comes in second in toddlers. (*p. 1709*)

12. **(d)** Legg-Clavé-Perthes disease occurs at a younger age. The pain is referred to the knee. (*pp. 1710–1711*)

13. **(c); 14. (a)** A classic history. (*p. 1705*)

15. **(d)** It is more important to recognize that the left tibia is abnormal than to recognize the disease entity (Blount's). (*p. 1700*)

16. **(c), (d)** Kyphosis and lordosis occur normally to some degree. (*pp. 1712–1716*)

17. **(e)** The onset is most often in adolescent girls. Neuromuscular and congenital forms represent 5% each. Idiopathic is 80 to 85% of cases. (*p. 1713*)

18. **(c)** The anomaly is phocomelia; the drug, thalidomide. (*p. 1691*)

19. **(d); 20. (b) and (d)** This is a classic history for dislocation of the radial head. Supination of the forearm is curative, and counseling parents not to pull small children by the arm is important. (*p. 1724*)

21. **(b), (d)** Ballet generally leads to hip and spine problems; football has head, neck, spine and limb injuries; gymnastic injuries are generally wrist, neck, and spine. It is baseball (especially in pitchers) and swimming that traumatize the shoulder. (*pp. 1728–1730*)

22. **(Salter-Harris 1 and 2); 23. (Salter-Harris 4); 24. (Salter-Harris 4 and 5); 25. (Salter-Harris 1)** "Ankle sprains" are often Salter-Harris 1 type fractures of the distal fibula. (*p. 1722*)

26. **(b)** Type I OI has the most constant blue sclerae. In other types, the hue fades in time. (*p. 1741*)

27. **(a), (d)** It is the proximal part of the extremities that is shortened; infants are hypotonic, although this resolves in time, and the bones are not demineralized. (*pp. 1732–1734*)

28. **(e)** The other name is Caffey disease, after the radiologist who first described it. (*p. 1745*)

29. **(b), (c), (d)** Children with Kneist dysplasia have sensorineural hearing loss, as do those with diastrophic dysplasia. (*pp. 1743–1745*)

30. **All are correct.** Other transient lesions include marmorata, harlequin color change, and transient neonatal pustular melanosis (*p. 1626*)

31. **(c)** Cavernous hemangiomas may disappear withsteroid treatment in some infants and are occasionally used in capillary hemangiomas in infants that are large and growing rapidly. Laser therapy will be best for (a) and (d). (*pp. 1629–1631*)

32. **(b)** In addition to melanoma, these nevi are associated with leptomeningeal melanocytosis. (*pp. 1633–1635*)

33. **(b), (d)** These vesicles are not infectious, pruritus does not occur, and steroid creams are not recommended. (*pp. 1639–1641*)

34. **(e); 35. (a); 36. (e); 37. (a); 38. (d); 39. (c)** The localization of the vesicle is of diagnostic and therapeutic importance. (*p. 1641—Table 23–3*)

40. **All these agents may cause contact dermatitis. (*pp. 1645–1647*)

41. **(b)** Pityriasis rosea is not hypopigmented, and the other choices itch. (*p. 1647*)

42. **All are correct.** When seborrheic dermatitis is intractable and associated with the absence of the fifth component of complement, it is known as Leiner disease. (*p. 1648*)

43. **(a), (b), (c), (d)** Lichen planus, but not lichen simplex chronicus. (*pp. 1649–1651*)

44. **(e)** The rash may also last from 2 weeks to 3 months. (*p. 1653*)

45. **(c)** Can be confused with (b), but responds to steroid treatment, which is not the case in tinea. (*p. 1659*)

46. **(a); 47. (c); 48. (d)** Toxic alopecia and alopecia totalis would tend to be more extensive. (*pp. 1666–1667*)

49. **(c)** Can be differentiated from herpes by its location on mucous membranes. (*p. 1669*)

50. **(a); 51. (b); 52. (b); 53. (c); 54. (a)** Ecthyma and blistering dactylitis are more severe forms of strep infection. (*pp. 1670–1673*)

55. **(a), (b)** These are the organisms that cause tinea versicolor and ringworm. (*pp. 1674–1677*)

56. **(e)** It is hard to see, but molluscum is usually umbilicated. (*p. 1679*)

57. **(c); 58. (a)** Treatment for scabes is best done with 1% gamma benzene hexachloride. Read, package insert carefully, especially for dosage in infants. (*pp. 1680–1682*)

59. **(b), (d), (e)** Diet is not a factor, and surface bacteria play no role. (*pp. 1683–1684*)

60. **(a); 61. (e); 62. (b); 63. (b), (c); 64. (d), (e)** An understanding of the basic principles of therapy outlined in the text will take some of the aura of witchcraft out of dermatologic treatment. (*pp. 1623–1626*)

65. **(a), (c), (e)** A dermatologist I know recommeds *never* using fluorinated corticosteroids on the face. (*p. 1625*)

23

Unclassified Diseases and Environmental Health Hazards

1. **(d)** The mechanism of death in SIDS is unknown, and the incidence is not increasing. Identifying "vulnerable" children will probably lead to neurotic parents, since the syndrome is not preventable, although some will disagree with this statement. SIDS excludes child abuse by definition, and vice versa, but a careful, competent investigation, done sensitively, is necessary to be sure of the diagnosis. (*pp. 1759–1761*)

2. **(c); 3. (a); 4. (b); 5. (d)** Sarcoidosis presents with these findings in very young children. Pulmonary findings occur in older children. Schüller-Christian syndrome presents with eosinophilic granulomas. (*pp. 1762–1766*)

6. **(c), (d), (e)** All radiation causes both biochemical and biophysical damage, and the less the tissue differentiation, the more the radiosensitivity. (*pp. 1769–1770*)

7. **(b); 8. (a); 9. (d); 10. (e)** Gonyaulax poisoning results from shellfish. Botulism wasn't listed in the symptomatology, but in infants will lead to weakness, poor suck, weak cry, and constipation. Honey has been implicated as the vector. (*pp. 1770–1774*).

11. **(a), (b)** The risk of aspiration is too great in a comatose (or semicomatose) patient, and alkali will corrode on the way up. (*p. 1776*)

12. **(a), (b), (c)** Alkalinization is useful for salicylate and phenobarbital poisoning. Neither alkalinization nor acidification helps remove iron. (*p. 1776*)

13. **(b), (d)** Infants and toddlers rarely suffer from acetaminophen toxicity. Methionine is no longer used, and hemodialysis is not effective. The Rumack-Matthew nomogram is used for plotting acetaminophen levels from 4–24 hours after exposure. (*pp. 1776–1777*)

14. **(a), (e)** Bleeding is rarely a problem in acute salicylism; the salicylate causes a metabolic acidosis by poisoning the Krebs cycle; and it is nonionized salicylate that is reabsorbed by the renal tubule. (*pp. 1778–1779*)

15. **(b), (e)** Tricyclic-antidepressants are most common. Alkalinization is useful only for long-acting barbiturates. Full recovery has occurred in barbiturate poisoning, even in the presence of a flat EEG. Pupillary signs are not of prognostic value. (*pp. 526, 1519–1521*)

16. **(b), (c)** Low-viscosity (high-volatility) hydrocarbons cause more damage, steroids are not of proven value, and fever and leukocytosis occur as a consequence of ingestion. (*pp. 1779–1780*)

17. **(a), (c), (d), (e)** A low serum level at 18 hours may be indicative of hepatic uptake and impending disaster. (*pp. 1780–1781*)

18. **(d); 19. (a), (c); 20. (c), (d), (e)** The case is one of imipramine overdose. The scenario is familiar, with the child hoping that if one pill might keep him dry at night, ten will do it for sure. It is not mentioned in the textbook, but better recognition of normally small bladders, and attention to subtler etiologies for enuresis (e.g., sexual abuse) could reduce flex prescription of imipramine. (*pp. 1781–1782*)

21. **(c)** Members of the arum family (Philodendron and Dieffenbachia) are chewed on most by children. Toxicity comes from calcium oxalate, reaction is local, and systemic manifestations are rare. (*p. 1785 — Table 26–3*)

22. **(c)** Also known as pink disease. (*pp. 1786–1787*)

23. **(a), (d), (e)** Rash and peripheral neuropathy are characteristics of mercury poisoning. (*pp. 1788–1791*)

24. **(b), (e)** Coproporphyrin and uroporphyrin are increased in the urine, whereas erythrocyte δ-aminolevulinate dehydratase levels are decreased. (*p. 1789*)

25. **(a), (c), (d)** The use of BAL is reserved for category III or IV lead poisoning, and D-penicillamine is not yet approved for use in lead toxicity. (*p. 1790*)

26. **(a), (b), (d)** Diethylstilbestrol administration in mothers is associated with carcinoma in female adolescent offspring, not birth defects. No teratogenic effects have been noted from dioxin in humans. (*pp. 1791–1792*)

27. **(c), (d)** PCB is found in breast milk, but at present the benefits of breast feeding outweigh the known risks. Asbestos is a problem when inhaled, but so far it has not been shown to be damaging when ingested. There is no evidence (in the textbook, anyway) that (e) is true. (*p. 1792*)

28. **(a), (b)** Supportive care alone will pull most humans through encounters with gila monsters, coelenterates, and stingrays. (*pp. 1793–1795*)

29. **(a)** Rabies is now rare, and *P. multocida* infection is an important but not most common complication. (*pp. 1795–1796*)

30. **(c)** The tarantula venom is not toxic to humans. The others are, although scorpions only give local reactions. (*pp. 919–920*)

You have now completed the questions in this book. That experience, plus 50¢, will get you a cup of coffee (or maybe you need something stronger). Nevertheless, you should retain something useful. On your next board exam you will know that the answers are not so: (b), (a), (d) . . .